Train Your Wandering Mind

COPE WITH ADHD
PERFORM BETTER AND FEEL BETTER

A book for Persons with ADHD or ADHD-like Issues

By

Michael Slavit

Board Certified in Cognitive and Behavioral Psychology

ISBN: 1505822289
ISBN 13: 9781505822281

Library of Congress Control Number: 2014922925
CreateSpace Independent Publishing Platform
North Charleston, South Carolina

Acknowledgements

—▬—

To my parents, Irma and Leonard Slavit,
for their love and support.

To my sister Betsy for her love, support
and skilled editing assistance.

To my sister Bobbie for her love and support.

To Dr. David J. Drum for years of guidance and assistance.

To Tom DiSanto for technical support and assistance.

—▬—

Contents

———

Concluding Chapter and References

Introduction

This book is not just for persons with ADHD.

THIS BOOK IS FOR ANYONE who has ever had difficulty maintaining focus while listening, reading, or doing tasks.

This book is for anyone who has ever looked around and found their surroundings too detailed or complicated to take in all at once.

This book is for anyone who has ever lost track of an important date or appointment.

This book is for anyone who has ever had problems misplacing items such as watches, keys, or cell phones.

This book is for anyone who has ever locked themselves out of their car, house or apartment.

This book is for anyone who has ever returned from shopping, only to realize that they have forgotten an item.

This book is for anyone who has ever been late due to losing track of time.

Michael Slavit

This book is for those who have ever felt frustrated with themselves for not being as effective, efficient and successful as they wished to be.

This book is for parents who are looking for ways to help a child to be better focused and organized.

(THIS BOOK IS FOR EVERYONE!)

———

Questionnaire

During your childhood, did you often experience the following:

1. Trouble sitting still in school?

2. School grades below abilities?

3. Trouble following classroom rules?

4. Trouble following rules in sports or games?

5. In frequent trouble with school authorities?

6. Difficult for parents to manage in social situations?

During your adulthood, have you often experienced the following:

1. Easily distracted?

2. Frequently lose things?

3. Make careless mistakes in your work?

4. Often late?

5. Often feel frustrated with yourself for being disorganized and forgetful?

6. Feel "on the go," as though propelled by a motor?

7. Sense of boredom when not directly stimulated?

8. Tendency to begin new tasks before completing earlier tasks?

9. Begin a day on one task and move on and on to successive tasks?

10. Frequent failure to make deadlines?

11. Inability to keep home, desk, or car neat and organized?

12. Tendency to not read through papers or documents?

13. Impulsive in making decisions before acquiring all needed facts?

14. Lack of interest in or tolerance for reading an entire book?

15. Tendency to allow others to provide facts or analysis?

16. Frequently interrupt others?

17. Blurt out answers before questions are complete?

18. Occasionally so focused on an activity that you fail to hear someone calling?

19. Usually feel your life is a constantly shifting maze of thoughts, plans and obligations?

20. Feel that there is an intelligent, competent person inside you, imprisoned by distractibility?

Thinking about the above items, have your problems with distractibility or impulsiveness ever caused you problems in the following domains?

DOMAIN	MILD	MODERATE	SEVERE
Health and Fitness			
Interpersonal Relationships			
School or Work Performance			
Control of Your Money			

The above instrument is designed as a stimulus questionnaire. There is no scoring system provided. If you have frequently had many of the experiences listed above, you may have Attention Deficit problems. For you to use this book effectively, it is not necessary to know whether you are considered to have diagnosable ADHD. Whether or not you have a diagnosable disorder, you probably have experienced a sense of disorganization and inefficiency. This may have resulted in inconvenience, and even embarrassment. There is no one among us who cannot benefit from working on improving our abilities to look at our obligations without becoming confused, to remain comfortable in the face of stimulating circumstances, and to keep our responses to life purposeful, organized and effective.

Read the book, with particular attention to the twenty methods described for improving your skills. If you are eager to get to the parts of the book that help you train your mind, and are less interested in some of the conceptual and scientific information, you may skip chapters 3, 5, 7 and 8, and still derive benefit.

———

CHAPTER 1
A Note about the Human Brain, Medication and About the purpose of this book

---

THE PURPOSE OF THIS BOOK is to help you develop your own inner resources. You will be taught ways to work on perception, cognition and behavior to overcome distractibility. This will improve your ability to live effectively, efficiently and successfully. The intent of this book is neither to encourage nor discourage the use of medication as part of your regimen to help yourself or your child.

In Chapter Eight, I will describe a tiny portion of the huge volume of research on this subject. One trend of the research has been to elucidate the link between the neurotransmitter amino acids dopamine and norepinephrine with ADHD. This is a critical area of investigation as it pertains to what has been the primary treatment of ADHD: medication. Most of the medications in use for ADHD - in particular the stimulant medications - are believed to exert their effect on these two neurotransmitters.

Michael Slavit

A Note on Perspective of Size and Number

The human brain is the most complicated system in the known Universe. You may have heard the old saw that there are as many neurons in the human brain as there are stars in the Milky Way galaxy. Well, that is not quite true. There are perhaps one hundred billion to two hundred billion, or even more, stars in the Milky Way. At last estimate, there are eighty-six billion neurons in the human brain. No one has actually counted all the stars in the galaxy or all the neurons in the brain. If you could somehow see all the neurons in a human brain, and could count at the rate of ten per minute, 24-hours per day, it would take you about 1500 years to count them all! Instead, a count is made in a very small volume. The percentage that that volume represents of the whole is calculated. Then the total is ascertained.

The average human brain has a volume of approximately 1200 cubic centimeters. Suppose that by using a staining technique that made the cell bodies show up, and by using an electron microscope, you could isolate one ten thousandth of a cubic centimeter of brain tissue. You might find about 7,200 neurons there. Since one ten thousandth of a cubic centimeter represents one twelve millionth of the whole brain, you could multiply 7,200 times 12,000,000 and calculate about eighty-six billion neurons in the entire brain. Why am I bothering to write this for you? To convey the message that with so many tiny structures, the size of the structures and the size of the connecting spaces between them - synapses - are extraordinarily small. What goes on at those small scales cannot be directly observed and is partly a matter of inference and conjecture.

The Neurotransmitters involved in Wakefulness and Attention

The following is a list of five of the neurotransmitters considered to be important in wakefulness and attention, and the brain areas that produce them.

Neurotransmitter	Brain Structure
Acetylcholine	Cholinergic nuclei
Serotonin	Raphe nucleus
Histamine	Tuberomammilary nucleus
Norepinephrine	Lucus coeruleus
Dopamine	Substantia nigra

Interestingly, only dopamine and norepinephrine have been consistently identified as targets of medications used in the treatment of ADHD.

Stimulant Medication
A long History of Non-prescribed Use

Most of the medications used to treat ADHD are stimulants. They are believed to act mostly by increasing the effectiveness of the neurotransmitters dopamine and norepinephrine, which are among the natural brain chemicals that are involved in activation, focus and motivation. A number of authors have asked the question, "Who would not improve their focus and energy when given a stimulant?" And, if fact, stimulants have been used without prescription for decades. Numerous sources have affirmed that professional baseball players have been using "greenies," a type of amphetamine, since 1970 or earlier. In addition, college and university students have been known for that same era to use Dexedrine to stay up late to write papers or study for exams. Whether or not one has been identified as having a disorder, stimulants temporarily increase wakefulness and focus. The question often asked, then, is "Do stimulant medications provide a remedy for an actual deficiency in persons with ADHD, or do they simply 'ramp up' the recipient's focus in the same way as they do so for a non-ADHD-identified person?"

PRESCRIBED STIMULANT MEDICATION AND THE TREATMENT OF ADHD

The first medication approved as a treatment for ADHD – Ritalin – was approved for this use by the Food and Drug Administration (FDA) sixty years ago in 1955. It was not until forty years later that other drugs were FDA-approved for treatment of ADHD. There are now at least twenty approved medications, though many of them are close formulations of one another, and some are extended release versions of the same medication. More than half the medications are stimulants. There are the amphetamine stimulants, such as Dexedrine, Adderall and Vyvanse. There are the methyphenidate stimulants such as Ritalin, Concerta, Metadate, Focalin, Methylin and Daytrana. An older atypical antidepressant – bupropion – is also used for this purpose, as are the blood pressure medications clonidine and guanfacine, and the non-stimulant medication Strattera.

In this book, Chapters eleven through thirty will teach you twenty methods to help you improve the ways in which you perceive your environment, think about your obligations and plan your activity. I strongly encourage you to read Chapters eleven through thirty carefully and experiment with the use of the suggested methods. The issue of whether to use a prescribed medication in addition to using these methods is not addressed in this volume.

CHAPTER SUMMARY

This book is medication neutral.

The human brain is extremely complex, and the structures within it are exceedingly small.

Stimulant medications have been in use on a non-prescribed basis for decades to enhance wakefulness, focus and performance.

The FDA-approved the first medication for treatment of ADHD in 1955 (generic name: methylphenidate; trade name: Ritalin). There are now over twenty medications in use, though many are very close formulations, or extended release versions, of others.

The stimulant medications in use for ADHD are believed to work primarily by enhancing the functions of the neurotransmitters dopamine and norepinephrine.

I will not suggest that you take medication for ADHD.

I will not suggest that you avoid medication for ADHD.

I will very strongly recommend that you develop your own inner resources, and work on the skills of perception, cognition and behavior to overcome distractibility. This will improve your ability to live effectively, efficiently and successfully.

In Chapters eleven through thirty, I will present a series of twenty methods for you to practice in order to achieve these goals. Chapter thirty-one is an illustration of an individual putting twelve methods to use in a single day.

Whether or not you take medication, you will do yourself a service by strengthening your own inner resources.

If you have a child with ADHD, you will do yourself and your child a service by helping your child to strengthen his/her inner resources.

———

CHAPTER 2
Positive Feedback Loops And Negative Feedback Loops

———

WE HAVE ALL HEARD THE expression, "Nothing succeeds like success." One interpretation of this saying is that success builds confidence, confidence leads to more success, and more success leads to greater confidence. This is an example of a positive feedback loop. Confidence and success may enhance one another repeatedly for a long time. I also refer to it as a "benevolent cycle." We have all heard about so-called "vicious cycles." For example, poor academic performance leads to poor self-confidence, which leads to worse academic performance, which leads to worse self-confidence, and so on. That is also an example of a positive feedback loop. That is correct. In this case, the words "positive and negative" are not the same as "desirable and undesirable." A positive feedback loop is simply one in which two phenomena keep one another changing in the same direction.

So, what is a negative feedback loop? It is a situation in which a change in one phenomenon causes a reversal of another phenomenon. You probably have a negative feedback loop in your home. It is called a heating system with a thermostat. As the furnace runs, the house becomes warmer.

However, unlike a positive feedback loop, the increased heat causes the thermostat to shut off the furnace, and the house cools down somewhat. When the house cools sufficiently, the thermostat turns on the furnace, changing the direction of the temperature and creating warmth.

Nature abounds with positive and negative feedback loops. For instance, consider the Earth's history from 2.5 million years ago until 11,700 years ago. The era is called the Pleistocene, in which much of the northern hemisphere was subjected to periods in which it was covered by vast ice sheets. These ice ages, or glaciations, were caused in part by positive feedback loops. The Earth grew cooler, perhaps due to changes in the degree to which the Earth's orbit is elliptical and the tilt of the Earth. As the temperatures grew colder, more ice formed. The increased ice then reflected more of the Sun's energy back into space, and the Earth grew colder, causing more ice to reflect even more of the Sun's energy back into space. That was a positive feedback loop.

This book is all about establishing desirable negative feedback loops and desirable positive feedback loops. You will be introduced to twenty methods to enhance your effective, efficient habits and behavior. The negative feedback loop I hope to help you establish is as follows. If you find yourself feeling disorganized and inefficient, you will experience emotional discomfort. Just as lower temperature in your home triggers the furnace to come back on and create warmth, your discomfort will trigger you to recall the techniques you have learned from this book. You will put the methods back into use, and your inefficiency and the feelings associated with it will reverse. That will be a desirable negative feedback loop.

As you strengthen your use of the methods you learned from this book, you will experience a renewed sense of self-control, which will cause your self-esteem to grow. Your enhanced self-esteem will feel so good that it will further strengthen your motivation to use the methods you have learned. That will be a desirable positive feedback loop.

After you have completed the book, it may be in your interest to re-read this section on positive and negative feedback loops. This may remind you to correct yourself if you have periods of slipping into less effective habits.

CHAPTER 3
The Power of One Organizing Principle

————

D O YOU KNOW HOW ICE forms from water? Before they freeze, water molecules are in constant motion. As long as the water molecules have sufficient motion, no ice crystals will form. When water does freeze, it does so quickly. You have probably witnessed this, perhaps to your dismay. For instance, you place a water bottle in the freezer, hoping to get the water to as nice, cold, and refreshing a temperature as you can. However, you do not want it to freeze. You check the water bottle occasionally, and see no signs of ice. Then, one time when you check it, the entire bottle has frozen. Why is this?

Water molecules freeze by arranging themselves in hexagonal patterns. Six water molecules form a hexagon and, as soon as one hexagon forms, the rest of the water molecules can quickly form more hexagons around the first.

If you have ADHD or ADHD-like issues, you can probably appreciate the idea that situations, obligations and expectations feel like water molecules in constant motion. Moreover, the idea of simultaneously arranging all those situations, obligations and expectations into an organized pattern may seem to be an overwhelming challenge. However, remember that not all the molecules of water have to freeze at once. Once one hexagon forms, the rest fall into place. Perhaps a similar pattern can help you in your battle to bring order and organization into your life. Start with one method to bring more focus and organization into one aspect of your life. You may be in for a pleasant surprise.

In this book, you will learn twenty methods to bring order and organization into your life. Relaxation training will be a great way to begin. After that, any one of the other methods may serve you in the same way that the first hexagon can serve a bottle of water.

CHAPTER 4
Use of this Book

———

*Strengthening your inner resources in an
enduring way will require practice and diligence
on your part. However, it is well worth it.*

THIS BOOK WILL PROVIDE YOU with specific methods to apply to the
problems of focus and memory, and to the maintenance of organized,
effective behavior. The methods presented are almost all internal techniques. That is, they involve the use of your own inner resources, rather
than the use of papers, calendars or electronic devices. The methods you
will learn will assist you in essentially building a stronger, more efficient
mental capacity.

One tenet of this book that will be repeated:

ADHD is not just something you are; it is something you do.

Moreover, if disorganized behavior is partly something you do, then
practicing methods to be better organized and more efficient is also something you can do. Whether or not you have an attention problem that is
diagnosable by accepted criteria, you can benefit. Almost all persons will

admit that, at least sometimes, they would like to be more effective, efficient and successful.

There is a chapter in this book entitled, *A Sampling of Research*. It did not seem appropriate to write a book about ADHD without at least some discussion of the multitude of research that has been done to study this topic. Much research has been done to look at brain structure. Researchers have studied the differences in structure between the brains of persons who have been identified as having ADHD and persons who are deemed to be developing normally. Researchers have used magnetic resonance imaging and other methods to study this issue. In addition, some researchers have turned their attention to an understanding of brain function. They have investigated the ways in which the various networks of nerve cells, distributed among different parts of the brain, combine to enable us to function.

You do not have to read the chapter on research to benefit from this book. This book provides practical methods you can apply immediately, without studying theory or research. If you wish to, skip the chapter on research and get right to the primary matter at hand: strengthening your inner resources.

There is another matter I want to re-emphasize. This book is medication-neutral. Whether or not to use medication for yourself or for your child is a matter for you to discuss with a physician who has expertise in understanding and treating attention deficit. No attempt is made in this book to encourage you to use medication for yourself or your child. No attempt is made to discourage the use of medication. However, I strongly encourage you to strengthen your inner resources, and I will give you specific ideas on how to do so. Whether or not medication is part of your treatment regimen, strengthening your inner resources is strongly encouraged.

There are twenty methods described in this book. You will undoubtedly not use all twenty. Read and consider all the methods presented. Start by practicing the methods that appeal to you the most, or that are most relevant to a specific issue you are experiencing. In time, it will be of benefit for you to try all the methods described. In the end, however, you will probably help yourself the most be retaining and practicing a selection of the methods that seem to work best for you.

Once you have made a selection of the methods that work best for you, it is your responsibility to practice them regularly. Coping with ADHD or ADHD-like issues is not like roofing a house. A new roof has a long duration. Depending on the quality of work and on the weather, you may not have to think about that roof for thirty years. Coping with ADHD is more like weeding a garden. Weeds grow back. Moreover, if you do indeed have ADHD, your tendency to lose focus, lose track of time, and to perform inefficiently may come back as well. Strengthening your inner resources in an enduring way will require practice and diligence on your part. However, it is well worth it. It is definitely and emphatically well worth it. Your efficiency and your self-esteem can take a huge step forward by applying the techniques described in this book.

———

CHAPTER 5
What is ADHD?
A Phenomenological Approach

———

THE PERSON WITH ADHD LIVES in a world in which, depending on the level of severity of his condition, the complexities of the world do not form patterns that he can see and sort out.

Phenomenology is the way in which one perceives and interprets events. You may think of it as referring to "the way in which phenomena make logical sense to an individual." Thus, in this section, I will endeavor to describe the way an individual with ADHD may perceive situations and events. For purposes of this illustration, I will describe ADHD as a condition in which the individuals have difficulty with the following:

1. differentiating between relevant and non-relevant details in a complex world,
2. assessing the relative importance of relevant details,
3. projecting oneself into the future, and
4. planning and executing coordinated responses.

Let us look at the first component: differentiating between relevant and non-relevant details in a complex world. The various types of stimulation that impinge on us – obligations, expectations, assignments, sights, and sounds – do not usually come single file. Imagine that you are about to leave home, with two destinations, and a total of seven stimuli. You want to stop at the post office to buy stamps, and to go to work. The weather report is predicting rain, and your umbrella is in the closet. Your favorite song is playing on the radio. Your work schedule will preclude going out for lunch, so you must bring your own. Your calendar shows your sister's birthday is in ten days. You will have to make an important work-related phone call, and the name and number of the person you need to call is on a 3X5 card on your kitchen counter. Those are seven stimuli: post office, work, weather, music, lunch, birthday and phone number. This array of stimuli can easily befuddle anyone. Six of the seven stimulus items are relevant. Only the favorite song on the radio is non-relevant.

Let us look at the relative importance of the six relevant items. Even though the sister's birthday is important, its relative importance is low as her birthday is ten days away. The post office stop is not very high in importance, as an errand of this type can be made later. Unless you have a condition such as hypoglycemia, your lunch is also of somewhat lower importance. This leaves getting to work, protecting yourself from the rain and making the important work-related phone call as the three concerns that are both relevant and important.

Projecting yourself into the future implies an awareness of the consequences of various choices. An efficient individual does not want to be late for work, arrive at work soaking wet, or be unable to make an important work-related phone call. Thus, an efficient, organized response would be to go back inside, grab the umbrella and the 3X5 card, and proceed directly to work.

However, what about an individual who has ADHD and has yet to learn appropriate coping mechanisms to combat the condition? Would he be able to see that the music playing is an irrelevant stimulus to be screened out in order to focus on the next task? On the other hand, would all the stimuli named appear to the ADHD sufferer to be like puzzle pieces scattered on a table with no apparent order? Unfortunately, for the person with ADHD, the latter might be true.

Even if the music were screened out as irrelevant, would the ADHD sufferer be able to assess the relative importance of the six remaining considerations – post office, work, birthday, rain, lunch, and phone call? Alternatively, would images of the six considerations swirl about in his head too quickly to apprehend them, sort them out and rate them? Again, unfortunately, for the person with ADHD, the latter might be true.

And, even if our ADHD sufferer had managed to decide that getting to work, getting there dry, and having the phone number were the three events that were both relevant and important, would he be able to get into and out of the house with the umbrella and 3X5 card quickly and efficiently? Or, would he either forget one of the two items, or be distracted by something altogether different and lose time on a tangential activity? Again, unfortunately, for the person with ADHD, the latter might be true.

The person with ADHD lives in a world in which, depending on the level of severity of his condition, the complexities of the world do not form patterns that he can efficiently see and sort out. It is as though he were suspended in a fish tank, with fish representing tasks, situations and obligations. Imagine that each approaching fish is different from the last one, moving quickly, and obscuring the view of the fish behind. How can you make sense of the world when it can appear that way?

Michael Slavit

Chapters eleven through thirty of this book will offer you concrete, easily learned methods to help you. You will be learning ways to perceive your world, think about your obligations, and organize your behavior in more effective ways. Moreover, your comfort, confidence and self-esteem will rise along with your improved efficiency.

———

CHAPTER 6
Disease, Disorder or Syndrome ?
A Matter of Definition

—▬—

DISEASE: A STATE OF IMPAIRED health caused by an invading pathogen or poison, resulting in an incorrectly functioning organ, structure, or system of the body and in pain, discomfort or impaired functioning.

Disorder: a state of impaired functioning resulting from the effect of genetic or developmental errors, nutritional deficiency or unfavorable environmental factors.

Syndrome: group of symptoms, without a specific, identifiable cause, that together form a characteristic pattern of behavior or action that may occur under certain circumstances and bring about discomfort or reduced functioning.

You will not *find* consensus about these definitions. For instance, the terms "disease" and "disorder" are sometimes used interchangeably. However, there are times when a distinction can be helpful, and I am advancing them for purposes of discussion and clarity. A few examples should serve to illustrate them.

Michael Slavit

If you were to be unfortunate enough to be bitten by a mosquito containing the microbe *plasmodium falciparum*, you would contract a serious disease called malaria. The symptoms are consistent patient to patient, and there is no doubt that the cause is the pathogen *p. falciparum*. This is clearly an example of a disease.

In 1943, fifteen years after its discovery, penicillin was introduced, and by the 1950's had become widely available as a remedy for certain infections. This includes the bacterium *staphylococcus aureus*, found on the skin and in the respiratory tract. However, there are few if any passive players in the game of evolution, and that includes microbes such as bacteria and viruses. By 1950, forty percent of hospital staphylococcus aureus isolates had evolved to a penicillin-resistant form. By 1960, this had risen to eighty percent. If you were to be infected by methicillin resistant staphylococcus aureus (commonly known as MRSA), you would have a specific disease caused by a specific pathogen.

Many of us have experienced a rash caused by contact with poison ivy. This rash is caused by sensitivity to an oily resin called *urushiol*, which is found in the leaves, stems and roots of poison ivy, poison oak and poison sumac. If you have ever experienced the intense itching with its resulting effect on your ability to sleep and concentrate, you would agree that your functioning is at least to some degree impaired. This impairment, the result of an identifiable environmental factor, would fit my definition of a disorder and not a disease or syndrome.

Another common disorder is gastro esophageal reflux disorder. This is a disorder in which the lower esophageal sphincter loses some strength or elasticity, allowing food and stomach juices to move up into the esophagus. This may cause a burning sensation commonly described as "heartburn," and can include coughing or even vomiting. Although it is sometimes referred to as esophageal reflux disease, by the definition I offer above it is a disorder and not a disease. It is more common among persons fifty years of and older, suggesting that the loss of resiliency of the lower esophageal sphincter is age-related. In addition, it can be caused by obesity or pregnancy. In addition, it can be caused by environmental factors such as over use of such foods and beverages as alcohol, coffee, fatty foods, chocolate, or peppermint. As this condition is not caused by an invading pathogen, but rather by habits or environmental factors, the term "disorder" is appropriate.

As to syndromes, two immediately come to mind: irritable bowel syndrome and fibromyalgia syndrome. Irritable bowel syndrome, or IBS, describes behavior of the digestive system. The term IBS is used when there is no anatomical abnormality or specific disease to which to attribute the gastrointestinal irregularities. Fibromyalgia is a particularly vexing situation, as some of the persons suffering from this syndrome experience very serious symptoms. There are theories about the origins of this syndrome but, as no actual anatomical abnormality or pathogen has been identified to date, it remains in the category of a syndrome.

HERITABILITY AND TWIN STUDIES AND THE CLASSIFICATION OF ADHD

Merriam-Webster dictionary on-line gives a simple definition of heritability: the proportion of observed variation in a particular trait (as height) that can be attributed to inherited genetic factors in contrast to environmental ones.

A way to determine if there is a genetic basis for a disorder is by studying large groups of identical and non-identical twins. Identical twins have the exact same genetic information while non-identical twins do not. Therefore, if a disorder is transmitted genetically, both identical twins should be affected in the same way. The probability of both twins being affected should be higher than that found in non-identical twins.

For common disorders, twin pairs will not always develop the same disease even if they are identical. This shows that these disorders are not completely determined by our genes.

To do a twin study under ideal circumstances, scientists must first make sure that they have identified all the twins in a given population. They must then find out how many have developed the disorder they want to study. In some countries, particularly in Scandinavia, all twins are registered at birth, which makes twin studies easier. As in all scientific studies, there can be some errors in the data collected from the twins. However, the main controversy is about how these data are interpreted.

If the likelihood of developing the same disorder is higher for identical twins than for non-identical twins, it is usually assumed that this difference is all due to inherited genetic factors. However, there is some dispute about whether it is possible to tell how much - if any - of this difference is truly due to genes. For example, if identical twins share more of the same environment or lifestyle factors than non-identical twins do, this could be an alternative explanation for any differences. Alternatively, if a combination of genetic and environmental factors interact to cause the disorder, this also reduces confidence in the calculated heritability.

There have been several major twin studies in past years that provide strong evidence that ADHD is highly heritable. They have had consistent results in spite of the fact that they were done by different researchers in different parts of the world. In one such study, Dr. Florence Levy and her colleagues studied 1,938 families with twins and siblings in Australia. They found that ADHD has an exceptionally high heritability as compared to other behavioral disorders. They reported an 82 percent concordance rate for ADHD in identical twins as compared to a 38 percent concordance rate for ADHD in non-identical twins.

We are certainly not aware of any pathogen that causes ADHD. A number of studies of the brain, using magnetic imaging techniques, have provided tantalizing, if not definitive, evidence that there is an issue of anatomical development. In particular, some research indicates that, while the brains of persons with ADHD develop with a normal structure, they do so with a delay. In addition, as discussed, studies of families and of twins have shown that there is a heritability factor. Thus, for purposes of our discussion, the term "disorder" appears to fit in the case of ADHD.

———

CHAPTER 7
Is the Definition Crucial?

There may be times when ADHD symptoms
are the final common pathway of anxiety,
personality factors and bad habits.

THERE IS NO DOUBT THAT many individuals have difficulty remaining focused, listening without being distracted, persisting with academic or work tasks, and managing their impulses. They can therefore suffer from reduced ability to succeed academically or occupationally, to live up to their obligations, to maintain positive health habits, to manage their money, and to relate to others without causing issues or resentments. These individuals need assistance in order for them to focus their attention, energies and behavior and to live more efficiently, effectively and successfully. They need assistance if they are to live effectively enough to experience self-confidence and self-esteem.

There is, nonetheless, a question as to the cause of these difficulties. I concluded Chapter Six with the statement that the term "disorder" appears to fit in the case of ADHD in that there is evidence of a delay in the anatomical development in the brains of persons with an ADHD diagnosis. However, there are undoubtedly many instances with alternative explanations for the problems of individuals identified as having ADHD. For instance, in my own practice I have often seen problems that I believed were the final common pathway of anxiety, personality factors and just plain bad habits. The type of assistance needed by individuals with problems with focus, persistence and impulse control may depend on the cause of their difficulties.

James Swanson and colleagues indicated that the precise status of ADHD is somewhat controversial. They state, "Some vocal critics even deny that this condition should be considered a disorder, citing the lack of clear evidence of a biological etiology." One of the most ardent critics of ADHD as a distinct diagnosis is Richard Saul, MD, who wrote a book, entitled *ADHD Does Not Exist*. In his book, Dr. Saul contends that ADHD does not actually exist as a separate disorder. Before you jump to any conclusions, be assured that Dr. Saul is sensitive to the issues of persons suffering from these problems. In fact, he states,

> It may often not matter whether ADHD is a disorder with an identifiable etiology. People have difficulties and need assistance. However, in some instances, it may make a great deal of difference whether ADHD is in itself a specific disorder. This would be the case in an instance in which attention deficit and/or impulsivity were symptomatic of another condition that could be treated.

> If there are other, underlying conditions that cause some individuals to experience issues in the attention deficit/impulsivity domain, then more needs to be done to help persons with these issues. Attention-related symptoms are all too real, with negative consequences for children, adults, and the broader society. Those affected face challenges in academic, professional and social settings, often with lifelong repercussions.

Thus, Dr. Saul is in no way ignoring the difficulties faced by individuals with problems with attention or impulse control. However, although he states clearly that these problems are "real and debilitating," he goes on to state,

> Over decades of clinical work, I have observed the multiple disorders and conditions that explain attention-deficit and hyperactivity symptoms.

Dr. Saul lists the following medical conditions that he believes can be responsible for attention deficit issues:

- Vision problems
- Sleep disturbance
- Substance abuse
- Mood disorders
- Hearing problems
- Learning disabilities
- Sensory processing disorder
- Giftedness
- Seizure disorder
- Obsessive-compulsive disorder
- Tourette's syndrome
- Autistic spectrum disorder
- Neurochemical distractibility/impulsivity
- Schizophrenia
- Fetal alcohol syndrome
- Fragile X syndrome
- Hyperthyroidism
- Pituitary tumor
- Other medical conditions (metal poisoning, iron deficiency, allergies, prematurity, or diet)

Let us consider, as an example, the first disorder on Dr. Saul's list: vision problems. Approximately half of the U.S. population has vision problems by adulthood and requires the use of vision correction by adulthood. Many children require assistance as well. In general, school systems are noted to be good at vision screening. However, what could happen to a schoolchild with an undetected vision problem? If that child were unable to read letters and numbers written by the teacher on the board, he or she might tend to look away and lose interest. The child would fall behind academically and, as the teacher had observed the child to lose attention and focus, ADHD might be incorrectly identified as the problem.

Sleep disorders are another category of issues that could be incorrectly attributed to ADHD. Sleep science has advanced very significantly in the past twenty-five years. We know that there are primary and secondary sleep disorders. Primary sleep disorders, relatively rare, are those disorders directly attributable to the functioning of the brain's circadian rhythm system. Secondary sleep disorders can be caused by a number of medical and psychological conditions. If a child were to be experiencing poor quality of sleep, the child would in all likelihood experience fatigue, and might well be distractible in school. Again, ADHD might be incorrectly identified as the cause of the child's school problems.

Vision and sleep issues are but two of the conditions that Dr. Saul believes are the actual culprits behind ADHD symptoms. If problems with attention, persistence and impulse control were in some cases part of the symptomatology of another condition, it would indeed in those cases be unfortunate if that other condition were not identified and treated.

In my own practice, I have frequently had patients come in for help with ADHD. As I previously indicated, after conducting my assessment, I have many times failed to detect what I considered to be true ADHD. I have at times informed the patient, and any referring party, that although the symptoms are present, they are in my estimation the final common pathway of anxiety, personality factors and bad habits. From my point of view as a psychologist, the treatment is the same, as you will read later in this book. The current volume provides assistance from a psychological and behavioral point of view. In this book, you will read about ways to use your own perceptions, thoughts and actions to perform more effectively.

I will close this discussion of whether or not ADHD is a disorder with quotations from the Institute of Mental Health. According to the 2012 revised edition of Publication No. 12- 3572 of the Institute of Mental Health,

> "Attention deficit hyperactivity disorder (ADHD) is one of the most common childhood brain disorders and can continue through adolescence and adulthood. Symptoms include difficulty staying focused and paying attention, difficulty controlling behavior, and hyperactivity. These symptoms can make it difficult for a child with ADHD to succeed in school, get along with other children or adults, or finish tasks at home."

The IMH report goes on to state,

> "Brain imaging studies have revealed that, in youth with ADHD, the brain matures in a normal pattern but is delayed, on average, by about 3 years. 1. The delay is most pronounced in brain regions involved in thinking, paying attention, and planning. More recent studies have found that the outermost layer of the brain, the cortex, shows delayed maturation overall. 2. brain structure important for proper communication between the two halves of the brain shows an abnormal growth

pattern. 3. These delays and abnormalities may underlie the hallmark symptoms of ADHD and help to explain how the disorder may develop."

Thus, according to the National Institutes of Mental Health, ADHD exists as disorder and has concomitants in brain development. With or without apologies to Dr. Richard Saul, we will accept that ADHD is a diagnosable disorder. However if, as Dr. Saul emphatically states, there are instances in which another diagnosable condition is present and is causing the difficulties, it may indeed be crucial to identify and treat the underlying condition.

——

CHAPTER 8
A Brief Sampling of Research

———

THERE IS A MULTITUDE OF research on the subject. Neuroscience has advanced very quickly during the past twenty-five years. This book will address summary conclusions of only a tiny portion of the enormous research information that has been reported. However, I will attempt to provide a flavor of a few of the trends of research. One trend focuses on the idea of differing ways in which subjects' brains integrate functions from different brain areas. Another focuses on structural and genetic differences in the brain. A third trend addresses the functional capacity of neurotransmitter amino acids such as dopamine and norepinephrine. In addition, a fourth trend addresses the question of how brain structure actually changes in response to the demands placed on it. Not all research efforts fall neatly into one of these categories, but I will try to list them in a relevant section.

INTEGRATION AND FUNCTIONAL CONNECTIVITY

Konrad and Eickhoff attempted to study both structural and functional connectivity in the brains of subjects with ADHD. They wrote, "Functional connectivity is defined as the temporal correlation or coherence of spatially remote neurophysiological events." I would like to draw an analogy to try to illustrate what Konrad and Eickhoff call "correlation or coherence of remote neurophysiological events." Imagine that your child has completed four successful years of high school. In the school office are records of your child's four years of accomplishments. Imagine that a violent tornado touches down, destroys the school's office, and lifts up, leaving the rest of the school intact. The tornado destroyed all computers and file cabinets in the office. You call the school superintendent and ask, "Are all the records of my child's four years of achievement forever lost?" The superintendent replies, "Perhaps not. I will send out a team to interview all the teachers. Some of your child's teachers from the earlier grades have gone on to other assignments, and it will take time to reach them, but we will try to re-construct the records." Within a few months, all teachers have been interviewed and, with a combination of their memories plus records they have kept, your child's record of achievement has been restored.

Does this not sound similar to the situation that arises when someone has had a brain injury or stroke? Some of the patient's functional abilities appear to have been lost. If you ask the doctor, "Are the patient's abilities forever lost?" the doctor will most likely reply, "It will be a while before we know. The brain is very plastic, and oftentimes other parts of the brain can take over the functioning of the damaged parts." And, in fact, within a few months, the victim of a brain injury or stroke may recover much or all of prior functioning. Part of the explanation is that many regions of the brain are involved in the creation and storage of memories and abilities, just as the memories and records of student achievement in our hypothetical example were retained by individual teachers. This attribute of brain function will probably prove to be relevant in the future as neuroscience reveals more about the causes of and best treatments for ADHD.

Although it seems to be widely accepted that various parts of the brain do work in concert, Konrad and Eickhoff described some of the difficulties inherent in studying these connections, and conclude, "Unequivocally acceptable assumptions are sparse." Konrad and

Eickhoff also indicated that there may be confounding environmental variables. For instance, ADHD subjects tended to have had lower birth weight, which has been linked to poor nutrition on the part of pregnant mothers. Mill and Petronis also reported that epigenetic processes may significantly influence development in ways that would affect susceptibility to ADHD.

In 2005 Katya Rubia and associates wanted to carry out a study that would eliminate the confounding effects of prior treatment with medication. She therefore studied adolescents who had been diagnosed with ADHD but who had never been treated with medications ("medication-naïve adolescents"). She used magnetic resonance imaging, and compared the adolescents with ADHD with a control group, and summarized their findings as follows:

"Rapid, event-related functional magnetic resonance imaging was used to compare brain activation in 16 medication-naïve ADHD adolescents and 21 IQ/age/gender matched healthy comparison volunteers during a challenging task. Results indicated that medication-naïve adolescents with ADHD showed significantly reduced brain activity in the right, inferior prefrontal cortex. The study shows that abnormal brain activation during ADHD is specific to the disorder, since it persists when medication history and performance discrepancies are excluded."

Sarah Durston reviewed imaging studies, and suggests that the idea of ADHD being primarily or exclusively a frontal lobe problem does not fit the data. She stated, "Posterior cerebral areas are also implicated in this disorder." Her research appears to be more in line with the concept of ADHD as an issue of integrating functions from different areas of the brain.

STRUCTURAL AND GENETIC DIFFERENCES IN THE BRAIN

Senior News Editor Rick Nauert, Ph.D. indicated that Researchers at Cardiff University School of Medicine and the University of Bristol in the United Kingdom do not believe ADHD is an either/or issue. Rather, they believe these issues exist in a spectrum – that there is a continuum in society of problems with attention, hyperactivity, impulsiveness, and language function. They suggest that there are clusters of genes that are associated with varying degrees of issues in the ADHD spectrum. Viewing these functions as existing on a spectrum based on the degree to which genetic factors line up is consistent with this author's definition of ADHD as a disorder as opposed to a disease or syndrome.

In the early 20th century, genes were thought of as immutable. It was not until Barbara McClintock began experimenting with maize (corn) that the stage was set for a change in this idea. McClintock observed genetic changes in maize in response to environmental stresses. In 1950 she published her first paper, "The origin and behavior of mutable loci in maize," describing transposable genes, now known as transposons, or "jumping genes." Her ideas were at first dismissed, and it took decades for this idea to be accepted. This is now known as the field of *epigenetics*, and it is now widely recognized that the genome can re-arrange itself in response to changes in the environment. Dr. Sharon Moalem describes this in detail in the book *The Survival of the Sickest*. We now know, for instance, that if a pregnant woman eats a lot of junk food during pregnancy, her developing embryo will sense that it is coming into a nutrient poor environment. The child will be born underweight and with a slow metabolism, a combination that would allow it greater survivability in a truly nutrient poor environment. Since the environment is actually calorie-rich, the child will be prone to obesity.

In addition, if a pregnant woman lives in a setting in which there is frequent crime, she may secrete a lot of adrenaline - the flight or fight hormone - into her blood stream. As she shares her blood supply with her unborn fetus, the developing child will do the same thing that its mother does: take blood from the brain and send it to the extremities. Thus, children who are born to mothers who resided in crime-ridden areas, or who ate junk foods, will be somewhat more likely to show signs of reduced brain development, and perhaps ADHD, as they mature.

Larry Seidman and colleagues studied the structure of the ADHD brain and concluded that the most consistently reported differences in the brains of children with ADHD were significantly smaller volumes in five brain areas. As indicated above, however, there may be environmental factors such as mothers' prenatal nutrition that may not have been accounted for.

James Hudziak and Stephen Faraone conducted a meta-analysis of four other studies with a total sample size of over one thousand. Although they asserted that ADHD has high heritability, they were nonetheless unable to identify any significant genome-wide associations.

Shaw and Ekstrand studied 223 ADHD-identified children and 223 controls. They used computational neuroanatomic techniques, and reported that they estimated cortical thickness at >40,000 cerebral points. They reported, "We found maturation to progress in a similar manner regionally in both children with and without ADHD. However, there was a marked delay in ADHD in attaining peak thickness throughout most of the cerebrum: the median age by which 50% of the cortical points attained peak thickness for the ADHD group was 10.5 years, significantly later than the median age of 7.5 years for the control group." This study is supportive of the position of the National Institute of Mental Health cited in the previous chapter.

Neurotransmitter Activity

ADHD and other similar conditions are believed by many to be linked to sub-performance of the dopamine and norepinephrine functions in the brain, primarily in the prefrontal cortex. A 2006 report from the Department of Neurobiology at the Yale University School of Medicine states, "The prefrontal cortex is very sensitive to its neurochemical environment, and optimal levels of norepinephrine and dopamine are needed for proper prefrontal cortical control of behavior and attention." The prefrontal cortex is responsible for self-regulatory function (for example, inhibition, motivation, and memory) and executive function (for example, reasoning, organizing, problem solving, and planning). There is some support for this hypothesis in the research literature. For instance, Karen Shue and Virginia Douglas tested children who had been identified as having ADHD as well as normal control subjects. While the subjects did not differ on tests of language (believed to be primarily a temporal lobe function), the subjects identified as having ADHD did more poorly on tasks believe to be representative of frontal lobe functioning

Due to variability in research methods, it has been difficult for a clear picture to emerge. Dawie Li and associates did a meta-analysis, comparing the results of published studies in European and Asian populations. Li concluded that there is an association between ADHD and dopamine system genes, though the nature of this association is unclear.

Brain Response to Demands

Bogdan Draganski and colleagues used magnetic resonance imaging to study the brains of medical students as they prepared for exams. They found structural changes in the posterior hippocampus as well as an increase in cortical grey matter. The hippocampus is the part of the brain that is central to short-term memory storage. There have also been studies of London Taxicab drivers. London is a particularly difficult city to learn, as there are no grids as there are in many U.S. western cities. Eleanor Maguire and colleagues have studied London cab drivers, and reported increased growth in the hippocampus. Other research shows that changes occur in brain structure and function in response to demands placed on it. This is cause for optimism. If demands are placed on the brain that force us to practice our ability to discern important patterns in the environment, focus our thoughts, and behave in an organized fashion, then perhaps we are having a direct and corrective impact on some of the causes of ADHD.

As you can see from this brief look, there is a considerable body of research reports in the professional literature. It is far beyond the purposes of this book to try to assess and analyze a significant portion of them. Perhaps the most tantalizing research results are those suggesting that the brains of children with ADHD are slow in developing. It does seem, however, that the recent emphasis on epigenetics may be decreasing the applicability of prior studies that did not account for these effects. In any event, from this author's point of view, the causes of ADHD may not be as important as are the methods used to treat it. People have difficulties and need assistance. This book provides assistance from a psychological and behavioral point of view. From this book, readers will learn ways to use their own perceptions, thoughts and actions to live more effectively.

———

CHAPTER 9
Train Your Brain

———

As human beings have invented more external memory devices,
we have exercised less of our ability to memorize.

Dr. Peter Jensen and many other researchers and practitioners have described the difficulty involved in sorting out the relative efficacy of medicinal treatment, behavioral therapy and combined treatments in the management of ADHD. Steven Safren and others studied adults who had been stabilized with medications but who were still symptomatic. They found that fifty-six percent of subjects who received cognitive-behavioral therapy (CBT) responded to treatment, compared to thirteen percent who did not received CBT. I will not specifically address this controversy in this book. However, studies such as that by Safren and his colleagues indicate that therapeutic outcomes are typically more effective when the individuals under treatment do not assume that salvation will come solely from a medicine bottle. Developing your own internal resources, or helping your child to develop his or hers, is extremely important if effective long-term adjustment is to be made.

Remember a basic tenet of this book: ADHD is not just something you are; it is something you do. This book will equip you with ways of improving your focus and organizing your efforts. You will be introduced to twenty specific ways of improving yourself from the inside. This book will not ask you to plan your time and tasks by the use of calendars, written lists, or to set up beeping noises by your hand-held electronic device. While those methods may have their place, the focus here will be on methods that will increase your internal strength and skill - to literally train your brain.

A very, very long time ago – before the advent of the printing press – a great deal of information was memorized, and was passed down generation to generation. This included practical life skill information, such as when to plant and harvest crops. But it also included stories, legends, and entire books. Information was stored internally – in memory. The inventions of writing, and later of the printing press, made such internal storage unnecessary. Information could now be stored externally.

A few decades ago, before the advent of hand-held electronic devices such as cell phones, people would typically memorize the telephone numbers of their friends, relatives, and other important numbers such as doctors' offices. Today, it appears that few people memorize telephone numbers; instead, they store the numbers in their hand-held electronic devices, and look them up when needed. This is very convenient, is it not?

However, there is a potential problem. As human beings have invented more and more external memory devices, we have exercised less and less of our ability to memorize. Memorization is not a simple trick. It requires use of a number of brain areas and a multitude of brain cells.

Have you had the experience of trying to recall some information, and having only partial recall? Of course you have. Perhaps you were trying to recall the name of an actor, actress, political figure, athlete, or fictional character. You may sometimes have remembered that it was a long name. You may have remembered the letter with which it began. You may have remembered that it was a common name, or an unusual one. What does this mean? It means that memory is complex. The memory of so simple an item as a name involves many, many bits of information. Because it is complex, memory requires a great deal of brain activity. As we have moved into an era that requires less memorization, we may be giving our brains less exercise. Just as physical exercise maintains our bodies in a condition that allows us to perform more activities, mental exercise helps us to maintain our brains in a condition that allows us to perform better mentally.

Again, a basic tenet of this book: ADHD is not just something you are; it is something you do. Some of the methods to which you will be introduced will help you to be less reliant on external memory and external devices, to improve your mental capabilities, to be more efficient and organized, and to feel better about yourself.

———

CHAPTER 10
Basic skill: Progressive Relaxation

———

Relaxation is not, in my opinion, a remedy for ADHD-like symptoms all by itself. However, it is an important basic skill that makes the other methods more effective.

CHRISTOPHER GILLBERG STATES, "ONE OF the most striking symptoms of ADHD is the difficulty in modifying one's activity level so that it is appropriate to the current situation." In order to modify one's activity level, one must first be attuned to monitoring it. Moreover, in the absence of experience with a quiescent state, such as a state of physical relaxation, monitoring one's activity level is a difficult, if not impossible task.

Relaxation is not, in my opinion, a remedy for ADHD-like symptoms all by itself. However, it is an important basic skill that makes the other methods more effective. The analogy I often use is that while long distance running is not by itself a soccer skill, being able to run distances is important for the acquisition of soccer skills. There are many ways to achieve physical relaxation, but the one I favor is a straightforward, clinical, no-nonsense approach called progressive muscle relaxation.

The method I will describe for you is called progressive relaxation. This method has been around, as far as the western world is concerned, since the early part of last century, when a physiologist named Edmund Jacobson devised it. Jacobson was a physiologist who worked at places such as Harvard, Cornell and Bell Laboratories. He was interested in what happens to people physically and medically when they say that they are nervous, tense and worked up. He and researchers since him have found some very interesting things. Every major system of the body is affected. The muscular-skeletal system is affected in that individual muscle fibers are shorter and tighter. Because those individual muscle fibers are shorter and tighter, there is increased activity in the nervous tissue that serves those muscles. Thus, the nervous system is affected. Because those individual muscle fibers are shorter and tighter, the muscles want more oxygen, so the respiratory system is affected. Since oxygen is delivered to the muscles through the bloodstream, the circulation system is affected. There is an increase in both blood pressure and heart rate. The endocrine system is affected, with an increased secretion of adrenaline into the bloodstream which, by the way, is a primary feature of a panic attack. The digestive system is affected, with an increased secretion of digestive acids. The integumentary system, which most of us call the skin, is affected in that there is an increase in skin conductance. And, some people get rashes like hives or eczema when they are tense. Even the immune system is affected. T-lymphocyte cells fight infection, recruit B-cells to further fight infection, and induce a cascade of reactions on the part of the human immune system. However, these immune system reactions are less active and less available when we are tense. In summary, every major system of the body is affected by physical tension.

To practice progressive relaxation, we first set aside fifteen minutes, and we find a place in which can be comfortable and in which we will be undisturbed for fifteen minutes. The very process of ensuring that we will be undisturbed can pay dividends. I have had adults tell me that insisting on fifteen minutes of undisturbed time changed the dynamics in their homes. Their children had to adjust to the fact that they were not the Centre of the Universe one hundred percent of the time. They learned that that Mom or Dad has needs and rights, too. All by itself, insisting on the time to practice relaxation is an exercise in reducing distractions and behaving more purposefully.

Progressive relaxation is such a fine technique that even a mediocre practice of it can have a desirable effect. However, I recommend having a well-refined, excellent way of practicing the technique. When we are first learning it, the technique takes about fifteen minutes. Jacobson wanted to find one of those physical changes that could come under some voluntary control, so he chose the shortening of muscle fibers. In order to lengthen the muscle fibers and to induce an array of other reactions, we first tense, and then release, muscles throughout the body.

Find a comfortable position in which to perform your relaxation exercise. If you lie down on a sofa or a bed, ensure that your back, neck and head are in a comfortably aligned position. If you are seated in a chair, make sure your feet can rest flat on the floor and that your hands and arms are in a comfortable and well supported position. Your next preparation for the exercise is to take a few slow, deep breaths, exhaling naturally. You want your abdomen to rise and fall with each breath. When your abdomen rises with an inhalation, your diaphragm descends, and your lungs can fill more fully. If you are not sure you are breathing in this way, place the palm of one hand on your abdomen and take a few breaths. Some people suck in their stomachs and expand their chests when they breathe. That is not as relaxing a way to breathe, and does not allow the lungs to fill as well with air. If you are in fact breathing that way, take a few moments to practice deep breathing with your abdomen rising as you inhale.

In our day-to-day lives we can become so involved with what is going on in our minds that we can totally lose touch with what is going on in our bodies. If you think about it, I am sure you will agree. Perhaps you can remember driving your car, and stopping for a break. Only at the break did you realize that you were driving all tensed up. Tension can build up without our even knowing it.

You are now ready to go through the body, one major muscle group at a time. When you put tension in, do not use all your strength or anything resembling it. Just put in a moderate amount of tension. And when you let the tension go, let it go all at once. You will go through your body one muscle group at a time. You will put in moderate tension, and will let tension go all at once. You will be taking a few slow, deep breaths, focusing your attention in certain, special ways and enjoying your resulting relaxation.

Begin with a slow, deep breath . . . . . and, let go. Again, take a slow, deep breath. . . and let go. Make sure that you are allowing your abdomen to rise and fall with each breath.

Now, remembering to use just a moderate amount of tension, make your right hand into a fist. Just be aware of what that tension is like, take a deep breath, and hold it . . . and, let go. Stretch your fingers out wide and, let them fall back into a natural, relaxed position. Your right hand may feel a little warm or tingly. Take a slow, deep breath. . . . and, . . . let go.

Same hand . . . make your right hand into a fist, and straighten your right arm, putting tension all the way to your shoulder. Take a deep breath, and hold it . . . . . and, exhale and let go. Stretch the fingers wide, and let them relax. Pay careful attention to the difference between the tight, tense feeling and the relaxed feeling. The more aware we are of the difference between these feelings the more easily we can let go ... and the more fully we can relax. Take a slow, deep breath ... and let go. Pause for a moment as you let yourself become fully aware of the difference between the tense feelings and the relaxed feelings. The next will be the last time for the right hand and the right arm. Make your right hand into a fist and straighten ... moderate tension ... hold it ... and, exhale and let go. Stretch your fingers out wide ..... and, let them fall into a natural position. Let your imagination help. Imagine any remaining tension draining down your right arm and out through the fingertips of your right hand.

Already you have learned a lot about how much tension you have to introduce in order for you to then fully appreciate, and fully enjoy, the feeling of relaxation. With that in mind, you will go to the left side. Do not introduce any more tension than you have to. Make your left hand into a fist. Put your mind and your awareness into that left hand and become fully acquainted with that tense feeling. Take a breath and hold it ... and, exhale and let go. Stretch the fingers ... and let them go.

With every muscle group that you work on you are going to feel more relaxed. With every muscle group you work on you are going to feel more calm.

Now make your left hand into a fist, and straighten your left arm. Introduce moderate tension all the way to the shoulder. Take a breath and hold it ... and exhale and let go. Stretch the fingers, and let them go. Be aware of what it feels like as the tension that you put in fades away. Be aware of what it feels like as relaxation takes over. Now this will be the last time for the left hand and the left arm. Make your left hand into a fist and straighten ... moderate tension ... take a breath and hold it ... and, exhale and let go.

Stretch the fingers . . . and let them relax. Notice the difference between tightness and relaxation. Just as with the right side, let your imagination help. Imagine any remaining tension draining down your left arm and out through the fingertips of your left hand.

Now draw your shoulders up as though you were going to pull them right up around your ears. Take a breath and hold it. Feel that tension . . . exhale, and let go. Let your shoulders enjoy the feeling that they are sinking down as deeply as they want to go. Let go a little more, and relax a little more. You will be surprised, and pleased, at how relaxed you can be. Make sure at this point that your hands and arms are in a comfortable, well-supported position.

In the muscles of the face you are going to introduce only a very small amount of tension – just enough for you to appreciate and enjoy the feeling of relaxation. We will start with the forehead. See if you can put a little tension in by gently knitting your eyebrows . . . and relax. Now gently raise your eyebrows . . . and relax. Feel what your forehead feels like as the tension that you put in fades away . . . and as relaxation takes over.

Now close your eyes and very slowly, very gradually, close your eyes a little bit tighter . . . and relax. You can allow your eyes to remain closed. Allow your forehead, your eyes, and your eyelids to all feel comfortable . . . perhaps a little heavy . . . and relaxed. Gently press your tongue against the roof of your mouth . . . and relax. Take a slow, deep breath . . . and . . . let go.

Place your teeth together in a good, firm, comfortable bite. Slowly, gradually, bite down a little harder, until you can feel some tension in your jaw . . . and . . . relax. As though you were very sleepy and had to yawn, open your mouth very wide like a big, wide yawn. And . . . relax. Allow your lips to remain a little bit apart, and feel what your face and your jaw feel like as the tension, and any tingling sensation that you introduced, fades away. Take a moment to notice the difference in the way you feel now compared to when you started.

Straighten your right leg, bringing your heel off the floor. Draw your toes back, stretching your calf muscle . . . and relax. Gently draw your right leg back just far enough for your foot to rest flat on the floor. Feel what your right leg feels like as the tension, and any tingling sensation that you introduced, fades away. Now straighten your left leg. Draw your toes back, stretching your calf muscle . . . and relax. Gently draw your left leg back, and feel what your left leg feels like as the tension, and any tingling sensation, fades away.

The last muscle group that you will add any tension to will be the abdomen. Take a breath and tighten your abdomen . . . hold it . . . and . . . exhale and let go. Continue to breathe normally. Be aware of what your abdomen feels like as it gently rises and falls with each breath. With every breath that you exhale, allow yourself to let go a little more. With every breath that you exhale, allow yourself to relax even more.

Think the following words: peaceful . . . calm . . . and serene. Imagine yourself saying those three words out loud . . . peaceful, calm and serene. You may find that you have a preference for one of the three. In your mind, select your favorite. And, in your mind only, without using your lips or your voice, think that word to yourself as you exhale. Do this for your next few breaths.

You have completed the tense/release portion of the relaxation exercise. The next instructions are for what I call "the focusing method." Draw your attention to your forehead and your eyes and let your forehead and eyes relax completely. Really let go throughout your forehead and eyes, and imagine the tiny muscles there becoming smooth and relaxed. Let your face and your jaw relax. Focus on a sense of stillness, like a pond without a ripple. Let your neck and your shoulders relax. Focus on a sense of letting go. And, as you let go throughout your neck and your shoulders, imagine the muscles there becoming smooth and relaxed. Let your right arm and your right hand relax, knowing, as you do now, that relaxation is a skill . . . knowing that you can acquire and then develop the skill of relaxation . . . knowing that in so doing you will be increasing your sense of self control . . . and knowing that increased self-control will improve your self confidence. Let your left arm and your left hand relax. Imagine any remaining tension draining down your left arm and out through the fingertips of your left hand. Let your entire upper body relax, including your shoulders, back and abdomen. Imagine tension leaving your body the way air might leave a deflating air mattress. Let the rest of your body relax, including your legs and your feet. As you each exhale each of your next few breaths, again, to yourself, repeat that word that you selected.

Imagine any remaining tension draining out of your muscles the way water might drain through a pipe, leaving your muscles smooth and relaxed. Let your shoulders feel that they are sinking down as deeply as they want to go, leaving your hands and arms heavy and relaxed. Focus on a sense of letting go, leaving you with a sense of stillness, like a pond without a ripple.

Continue to relax for a few more moments, and tell yourself the following:

- At this moment you have no obligations other than to relax.

- In the week ahead you will retain a clear memory of the way you feel now, and even that memory will help you.

- Every time you practice relaxation you will succeed, and you will become more skilled with practice. If you relax before sleeping, you will sleep more peacefully and therefore, of course, you will awaken more refreshed.

- Even more importantly, if you relax soon after rising, it will help you begin your waking period more relaxed. That will make you so much more aware of what tension feels like at its earliest noticeable onset, that you may be able to prevent its build-up in the first place. That will be a great accomplishment, and a savings of energy – energy that would otherwise be squandered in nervous tension.

- Something will happen this week . . . something that might ordinarily make you feel nervous or rattled. But you will feel less nervous than usual. You will deal with it. You will find a solution. You may even feel that you have shed a bit of unpleasantness from about you the way you would shed rain from an umbrella. And that will feel good.

- When you conclude the exercise and open your eyes, you will still feel relaxed, and you will also feel alert, refreshed, and with a sense of well being. You will also be very much aware that you can develop your own internal skills to help yourself.

That concludes the progressive relaxation exercise. You may want to read the entire description as it is written on these pages before performing the exercise, and then to do the exercise by memory. A second method would be for you to read the transcript aloud and to record it for yourself. You would then be able to play it back for yourself as you perform the exercise. A third method would be to have another person read the instructions for you as you learn the technique. Regardless of which way you choose to acquire the skill of relaxation, you will find deep relaxation to be an enormous help in quieting your body and mind in such a way as to set the stage for more organized thought and actions. The next two pages are a brief review of the recommended use of the progressive relaxation method that has been described.

Review of Progressive Relaxation

Since relaxation and anxiety are incompatible states, you can reduce anxiety by developing your ability to experience deep relaxation.

Set aside 15 minutes, and try to ensure you will be left undisturbed.

Sit comfortably in a chair, or recline, or lie down. If you sit up, place your feet flat on the floor and be sure your hands and arms are comfortably supported. If you are reclining or lying down, be sure your head, neck and back are comfortably aligned.

Experience the difference between tense and relaxed feelings by tensing and then relaxing muscles, as has been described. Introduce only as much tension as you need. After you have applied tension, take a breath and hold it for 3-5 seconds. Let go of tension all at once, as you exhale your breath. Do not hold your breath while working on the muscles of your face and head. Apply this procedure to your hands, hands and arms, shoulders, forehead, eyes, tongue, jaw, legs and abdomen.

After releasing tension, take a few moments to really feel and appreciate the difference between tense and relaxed feelings.

THE FOCUSING METHOD: Draw your attention to each muscle group again, one at a time. This time introduce no tension. Rather, just allow relaxation to deepen in one of the following ways:

- Imagine your muscles becoming smooth and relaxed.
- Imagine tension draining out of your muscles, like water through a pipe.

- Imagine tension leaving your body the way air might escape a deflating air mattress.
- Just focus on a sense of letting go.

Now and then, throughout the exercise, take a slow, deep breath and let it go. As you exhale, think your choice of the following three words: "peaceful, calm, or serene."

Practice these exercises three times per day. The purpose of these exercises is to build your skill of relaxation – not just to help soften a stress-filled week. Practice the exercise regardless of whether you are having an easy or a difficult week.

In the next chapter you will next read instructions on how to create a brief relaxation method. In order for the brief relaxation method to be optimally effective, it is important that your body and mind truly learn the deep sense of relaxation that you experience with the full relaxation method. Ideally, you would practice the full relaxation method three times per day for a week or two.

———

CHAPTER 11
Method One
The Brief Relaxation Method

——■——

HAVING LEARNED AND PRACTICED THE full relaxation method, you are ready to acquire a brief method. Start by putting yourself into a relaxing situation, just as when you learned the full relaxation method. Then, take a few slow, deep breaths, thinking to yourself the word you selected previously (peaceful, calm or serene). Now, read each the following eleven instructions, taking fifteen to twenty seconds after each to sense its effect on you:

1. Just focus on a sense of letting go.

2. Imagine tension draining out of your muscles, the way water might drain through a pipe.

3. Imagine tension leaving your body the way air might leave a deflating air mattress.

4. Let your shoulders enjoy the feeling that they are sinking down as deeply as they want to go.

5. Imagine your muscles becoming smooth and relaxed.

6. Imagine your muscles becoming warm and relaxed.

7. Imagine your muscles becoming soft and relaxed.

8. Just focus on a sense of stillness - like a pond without a ripple.

9. Imagine your hands and arms feeling heavy and relaxed.

10. Imagine the sensation of floating.

11. Focus on a sense that a burden has been lifted from you.

Next, make a selection of the four or five of the eleven focusing methods that you feel have the greatest relaxing effect on you. Then, carry out a series of experiments. Each experiment could take about twenty seconds. Take a slow, deep breath, and think your favorite word ("peaceful, calm or serene") as you exhale. Then let yourself experience two of the focusing methods.

Thus, your method may be like any of the following:

"Take a slow, deep breath . . . think 'peaceful' as you exhale . . . focus on a sense of letting go, and on a sense of stillness, like a pond without a ripple."

"Take a slow, deep breath . . . think 'calm' as you exhale . . . let your shoulders sink down as deeply as they want to go, leaving your muscles smooth and relaxed."

"Take a slow, deep breath . . . think 'serene' as you exhale . . . imagine tension draining out of your muscles, the way water might drain through a pipe, leaving you with the sensation of floating."

As there are eleven focusing methods. The first can be any of eleven, and the second can be any of the remaining ten. Thus, there are 11 X 10 = 110 possible permutations of two focusing methods. As these selections of focusing methods may be combined with any of three words, there are, in total, 3 X 110 = 330 possible brief relaxation methods. Do not worry about finding out which of the 330 possible methods is the very best for you. Just experiment with a small number of combinations, and select one with which you feel comfortable, and that has a noticeable effect on your state of arousal when you use it.

In your daily life, there will be situations in which you feel the total stimulation you are facing is overwhelming your ability to sort out that stimulation. When you sense this, pause for twenty seconds to perform your brief relaxation method. If needed, repeat it another time or two until you feel less tense, less aroused, and better able to sort through the stimulation in front of you.

—■—

CHAPTER 12
Method Two
Stop-Scan-Do

———

ADHD CANNOT BE CURED, BUT we can develop coping skills to alleviate its effects. Keep in mind that practicing a self-administered method to cope with ADHD is not like roofing a house. It is more like weeding a garden. When you roof a house, you do not have to think about the roof for 25-30 years. However, weeding a garden is a daily task. Coping with ADHD is a daily or even a moment-to-moment task as well.

This method is at the same time a very simplistic and yet profound method to combat ADHD. I call it "Mindfulness-based Self-administered Regulatory Protocol." Actually, I do **not** call it that. I call it "Stop-Scan-Do."

Almost all of us have had two or more demands on us at the same time, and have felt as though we were literally being pulled in different directions. We have essentially felt immobilized – suspended between or among demands. You may employ the stop-scan-do method to avert those experiences, and I can best explain it with illustrations.

Michael Slavit

Picture an individual making a breakfast consisting of a fried egg, toast and tea. He puts the whistling teapot on the stove and puts a high light under it. He then puts a piece of bread in the toaster and pushes the lever down. Then, as he is getting an egg and some butter or margarine from the refrigerator, and getting a fry pan from storage, he realizes that the toast will be cold if he lets it finish toasting now. As he turns to stop the toaster, he realizes the water is boiling and the teapot is whistling shrilly on the stove. He has to stop the toaster . . . no! the teapot . . . no! the toaster . . . . . no! the teapot. He is suspended between these two demands, as though one person were holding his left outstretched wrist and a second person were holding the right. Most importantly, he is feeling frazzled, tense, and incompetent.

Let me illustrate how this breakfast preparation might go using the stop-scan-do method. Our hypothetical cook places the teapot on the stove with no flame under it. He places the bread in the toaster without pressing the lever. He places the fry pan on the stove with no light under it, and places the egg and butter nearby. He stops and scans. (Scanning implies a quick assessment of the situation). He knows he does not want cold toast, so he does not press the lever. Instead he puts a medium flame under the teapot and he scans. He still does not want cold toast, so he places a pat of butter into the fry pan and he scans. He hears sounds from the teapot indicating the water is heating up, so he lowers the flame to low, and he scans. He still defers starting the toast, so he places a high flame under the fry pan, and he scans. The butter is beginning to melt in the pan. He cracks the eggshell and drops the egg onto the pan, gets the egg skating on the pan, and turns the flame down to low, and he scans. It is time to push down the lever on the toaster. He notices that the teapot is beginning to whistle gently, so he turns off the flame and pours the water into his teacup. In a moment, the egg appears done, so he slides it onto a plate, just as the toast pops up. He has a hot egg, hot toast and hot tea. It all came together efficiently. However, most importantly, he is relaxed, and he never felt tense and frazzled. He never felt suspended between demands.

Have you ever found yourself in the awkward position of holding in your hands the tools for a task, and realizing that you have to put them back down and attend to a task that should have preceded it? An example would be holding a paintbrush, wet with paint, and realizing you had not yet positioned the object to be painted. Another example might be holding a screw and an electric drill, and realizing you had not yet plugged in the drill. The minor problem is that you are temporarily inconvenienced, and use extra time. The major problem is that you may criticize yourself and define yourself in negative terms (for example, "I am a space shot" or "I am such an airhead"). Using the stop-scan-do method will help you to sequence the steps to your tasks more effectively. Then, you can define yourself in much more positive ways, and you will feel much better about yourself.

It will be important for you to use your imagination and think about as many situations as you can in which the stop-scan-do method may be helpful. Then make mental pictures of yourself implementing the method in those situations. This will help you to remember the method when the situation does arise. The important point is that you need to understand the concept, and you have to be motivated to look for situations in your life in which you can apply it.

CHAPTER 13
Method Three
The Internal Monitoring Method

———

W E HAVE ALL EXPERIENCED THE nagging feeling that we are forgetting something – that there is some obligation that we are not meeting. The feeling itself can detract from our ability to be fully present and to enjoy ourselves. In addition, there may be a situation or obligation that does, in fact, require our attention.

The internal monitoring method is a technique we can apply with a few minutes of time and some concentration. It does not require a calendar, cell phone, or other electronic device. I introduce patients to the method in session. On the other hand, you will have to teach it to yourself after reading this description. It is helpful to begin with a moment of relaxation to help minimize distractions. After relaxing, we bring our attention, one at a time, to six different areas of life activity. When we think of each category, we first assess how we are feeling about that sphere of our life. Secondly, we identify anything that we would prefer to attend to or to improve in that domain. Thirdly, we identify in our mind the first, achievable step we can take to improve that part of our life. Lastly, we identify the time when we will be able to take that first, achievable step.

We briefly return to relaxation in between thinking about the different spheres of life. Repeat this procedure for each of the areas of life activity listed below. When you have identified concerns to which you want to attend, remind yourself that you have not signed a contract or made an irreversible commitment. You have simply identified steps toward improving six areas of your life, and have decided on a time when those steps may be taken. Alternatively, you may have solved that little puzzle of the nagging sense that there is something forgotten. The goals and the steps toward the goals can always be changed, or even ignored.

- Material / financial
- Recreational / physical
- Social
- Home / domestic
- Intellectual / spiritual
- Professional / vocational

To remember these categories, use the memory device "MR SHIP."

M - Material
R - Recreational
S - Social
H - Home
I - Intellectual
P - Professional

This method will help you if you have sometimes forgotten an obligation. Periodically, throughout your day, you may want to bring your attention, one at a time, to these six types of obligations. If you find it difficult to do so, you can train yourself to use this method at specific moments – moments when you have or are about to perform a typical function. For instance, you could review "MR SHIP" at any of the following times:

- After having morning beverage
- Before leaving house
- Before resuming activities after lunch
- Before leaving work

In addition, review "MR SHIP" whenever you have a nagging feeling that you may be forgetting something. By reviewing these six categories of life obligations, you will often avoid the experience of failing to attend to an obligation. You will replace feelings of being scattered or disorganized with feelings of being clever and competent. There will be both practical and emotional benefits, and your self-esteem will surely rise.

———

CHAPTER 14
Method Four
RCA-V

———■———

THIS IS AN EXTREMELY SIMPLE method to help overcome a problem common to many individuals, whether they are identified as having ADHD or not. Many persons complain that when they leave one location for another, they either leave something incomplete and/or they forget to bring something they need for their next assignment.

RCA-V stands for "RCA Victor," a commercial insignia with which most people are familiar. You probably recall an insignia with a dog sitting beside an old-fashioned phonograph. There is no significance to the name; it is merely a memory device.

Very simply, RCA-Victor is intended to help you go through the following steps when you realize they are about to leave one location for another.

R   **Relax** (use the brief relaxation method)

C   **Complete** what you were working on, and put away any items needing to be stored.

A   **Attend** (to what you need for your next assignment), and

V   Velocity (**Go!**)

As simple as this method is, it can save you great inconvenience. By beginning with brief relaxation, you will reduce your overall arousal level. As previously discussed, making sense of the complexities of your environment becomes easier when your arousal level is reduced.

The next step is completing what you were engaged in, and putting away any items needing to be stored. This has a number of distinct advantages. It makes your experience easier when you return to that setting. It also reduces the likelihood that other persons will judge you to be disorganized and inefficient.

Then, the method suggests that you attend to what you need for your next assignment. There is no one among us who has not arrived somewhere, only to find we have forgotten to bring an important item. It could be water, food, a gift, warm clothing, an umbrella, an admission ticket, a picture ID, athletic equipment, money, checkbook, or any one of innumerable items. In order to make sure you have the needed items, picture yourself, as in a movie, arriving at your next assignment and taking part in your activities there. If you make a careful enough picture of your next assignment, it is likely you will identify the items you need.

The fourth step is "velocity" – go. Try to develop the habit of engaging this quick sequence before leaving one location for another: R – C – A – V.

CHAPTER 15
Method Five
Acronym for Remembering

—■—

Persons with ADHD frequently complain about their memory for day-to-day items. They are often self-critical, and are often subjected to criticism by others.

Many years ago, when I was a college undergraduate, I served as the head lifeguard at a swim and tennis club. I had various responsibilities, including locking up the club at night. Another responsibility had to do with the system we used to chlorinate the swimming pool. We used a liquid chlorine that was fed into the pool's filter through a long tube, which I termed a "leader," for a reason that will soon become apparent. The chlorine feed had to be shut off for the night. When I locked up the club and left for the night, the door by which I left was at the back of the kitchen, which I referred to as the "larder," for reasons that may be dawning on you. I had to make sure I had taken the first aid kit and a few other items from the lifeguard chair, which I termed the "ladder," for reasons that must now be obvious. In addition, I had to make sure my own locker was locked.

Michael Slavit

One morning I came in and discovered that when I left the night before I had not unhooked the chlorine feed (the "leader"). I panicked. I checked the chlorine level in the pool, and it was very high. Fortunately, it was a very sunny day. Sunlight causes a breakdown of the chlorine formula in the pool, and the chlorine level returned to normal soon. However, I was determined not to make a serious mistake again. I thought about my end-of-the-day responsibilities, and came up with the following mnemonic device:

L   Locker (lock my own locker)
L   Leader (unhook the chlorine feed).
L   Ladder (be sure the first aid kit was off the lifeguard chair)
L   Larder (be sure the kitchen door was locked on departure).

When I was Director of Counseling at Southern College of Technology years ago, I had a client who diagnosed herself as having ADHD. She complained that she was very forgetful, and that her husband was critical of her for some of her errors and omissions. For instance, she would often leave for work and leave on the air conditioning (or heat, depending on the season). She would forget her lunch, her purse and her keys. When she forgot her keys, she would have to call her husband, who was displeased at having to leave his work early to go home to let her back into the house. She would make very self-deprecatory comments, such as, "I'm such a space shot." After a little thought, I gave her the mnemonic "P-L-A-K":

P   Purse
L   Lunch
A   Air conditioning (or heat, depending on the season)
K   Keys

I instructed her to teach herself to think "P-L-A-K" every time she left her home. She quickly learned the memory device, put it to use successfully and, voila, she was no longer a "space shot." She felt much more confident and reported better self-esteem. We did not have to work through any childhood experiences or feelings. We did not have to do anything lengthy or complex. She came in with a self-esteem issue that was specific to certain episodes of forgetfulness, and we dealt with it with a simple memory device. I have made literally scores, and perhaps a hundred, of these simple devices for patients over the years, and in most of the cases the patients do in fact teach themselves to recall their mnemonic, and they typically report success.

—◼—

CHAPTER 16
Method Six
Cognitive Mapping

———

People who frequently forget about or are late
for appointments or other obligations quite
likely have poor cognitive maps of time.

WHAT IS A COGNITIVE MAP?

A COGNITIVE MAP IS AN INTERNAL representation of some aspect of the
world – usually a picture of locations, time, or both. A cognitive map
may be a direct representation, such as a mental picture of the rooms in
your house or apartment, or of the streets in your neighborhood, just as
they are. Or, they may be your own individualized internal maps, without
any direct relationship to the part of the world you are representing.

DO WE ALL CREATE COGNITIVE MAPS?

The probable answer is "yes." We would have a hard time indeed finding
our way through life – both in terms of time and space – if we did not
have an internal representation of the world we are navigating. However,
people vary greatly in the skill and accuracy with which they create their
internal representations of the world. This probably accounts for why

some individuals are so much more likely to become lost, or be late for appointments and obligations. They simply lose track of where they are – either physically or with respect to the time.

CAN I IMPROVE MY SKILL AT MAKING COGNITIVE MAPS?

Yes, just as with most other skills, this is one you can work on and improve. First, you may want to figure out what some of your cognitive maps look like. Remember, your internal representations of the world may be vivid, or indistinct, or you may be unable to detect them at all.

COGNITIVE MAPPING OF TIME

Do you have a picture in your mind of the months of the year? Perhaps you have one of which you are quite well aware. Perhaps you think you may have an indistinct one. Alternatively, perhaps you are unaware of having any visual representation of the months of the year.

The following is one person's cognitive map of the months:

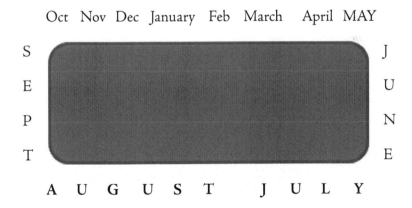

Michael Slavit

It should be obvious that for the owner of this cognitive map, summer is, or was, very important. In fact, this individual formed this map during childhood, during which time his family had a summer home. Summertime was so important to him that, to this day, July and August appear as large as October through May in his conceptualization of the months of the year. June and September appear as "wrap-around months," making the transition from spring to summer and from summer to fall.

How about you? Does this example awaken in you any realization that you, too, have some kind of picture of the months of the year? You probably have one, though it may be vague or indistinct. And you may not be consciously aware of it. However, if you can bring it more consciously to mind, it can help you to remain aware of the plans and obligations that are relevant to the present time.

One person's very simple cognitive map of the days of the week is a long rectangle going from left to right. It is divided into eight boxes. Why does he see eight instead of seven? This individual sees a separate box at the far left for Sunday night. Essentially, in his mind, his weekend ends a little early, and Sunday night is seen as a separate time to prepare for the week ahead.

Sunday Night	Mon	Tues	Wed	Thurs	Friday	Sat	Sun

Here is another map of the days of the week:

MON	Tues	Wed	Thurs	Friday	Sat	Sun
6:00 am	6:00 am	6:00 am	6:00 am	6:00 am	6:00 am	6:00 am
Noon	Noon	Noon	Noon	Noon	Noon	Noon
6:00 pm	6:00 pm	6:00 pm	6:00 pm	6:00 pm	6:00 pm	6:00 pm
Midnight	Midnight	Midnight	Midnight	Midnight	Midnight	Midnight

This individual seems to see each day as divided into the three parts of morning, afternoon and evening. There does not seem to be a space for midnight to six a.m., so we can surmise that this individual keeps regular hours and does not consider the wee hours of the morning to be part of his life worth mapping.

It is quite likely that these cognitive maps are not as one-dimensional and sterile as they appear on these pages. Imagine that, associated with each of the blocks of time depicted in these maps, there are pictures relevant to plans and obligations that we expect will occur during the time blocks. There may be pictures of places such as classrooms, athletic fields, office buildings, supermarkets, doctors' offices or beaches. There may be pictures of people – either individuals or groups. The pictures for most persons are probably not distinct and vivid. They are most likely faint and ephemeral, changing as our thoughts and plans for our days, weeks and months change. The point is that for most persons these internal representations of time blocks, and the pictures associated with them, do exist, and they help us to remain aware of our plans and obligations. Cognitive maps enable us to keep track of, and therefore to be responsible for, upcoming events in our lives.

ARE THERE PEOPLE WHO HAVE POOR QUALITY COGNITIVE MAPS?

I think the answer to this should be obvious. People who have difficulty finding their way to places they have visited probably have not developed good cognitive maps of space – of roads, bridges, or paths. Moreover, people who frequently forget about or are late for appointments quite likely have poor cognitive maps of time. I have become aware that many persons who are identified as having ADHD have very poor, and sometimes virtually nonexistent, cognitive mapping skills. However, it is possible to consciously create cognitive maps and to practice using them to your advantage.

COGNITIVE MAPS AND THE EARLY DEVELOPMENT OF ARITHMETIC SKILLS

Many people have difficulty with mathematics, and this probably has its roots in very early arithmetic skills. When prospective patients call me and identify themselves as having ADHD, I often give them the following problem:

Imagine you are looking at a field. There is a fence running right down the middle of the field. On the RIGHT of the fence are THREE sheep, and on the LEFT of the fence are TWO sheep. How many sheep are there in all?

The people always correctly answer "five." I then ask them to subtract 68 from 73, and they almost always become flustered. "Um . . . . . let's see . . . . . 8 from 3 . . . no, I can't do that . . . . . let's see . . . . . borrow the one . . . . . . I'm not good at math."

I then ask, "You easily know that THREE sheep on the RIGHT of the fence plus TWO sheep on the LEFT of the fence equals FIVE sheep. How is that any different from seeing that 73 minus 68 equals five? The number 68 is TWO steps to the LEFT of seventy and 73 is THREE steps to the RIGHT of seventy.

| 65 | 66 | 67 | 68 | 69 | **70** | 71 | 72 | 73 | 74 | 75 |

If a person can imagine a number line, with more pronounced lines for multiples of ten, then many arithmetic calculations can easily be made. It is very possible, and in my view quite likely, that the lack of good cognitive mapping is often a factor in the existence of early difficulties in arithmetic skills.

HOW MANY WAYS ARE THERE TO USE COGNITIVE MAPS?

The use of cognitive maps is probably limited only by the limits of your imagination. You may use cognitive maps:

- To keep track of your obligations during a day;
- To keep track of your obligations during a week;
- To recall the route to an important destination;
- To retain and recall the points you want to talk about in a speech or presentation;
- To make arithmetic calculations;
- To learn and retain the components of an electrical circuit;
- To remember the ingredients of a favorite recipe;

Pick out a set of tasks or obligations that are important to you and in which you would like to make improvements. Next, experiment with ways in which you can make internal representations of a time period that will help you to be more effective in managing these tasks or obligations.

Get ready for some hard work, and do not give up! When you first attempt to construct cognitive maps, you may encounter difficulty.

Think about a time period ahead of you, and make a visual representation of that time period. Make sketches of some of your ideas with pencil and paper. When you have sketched something that seems promising to you, look at it for several seconds and then close your eyes and try to visualize it. Next, think about your obligations for the time period. Make some images in your mind of the places you will be, the items you will use or the persons you will encounter. Place these images in their appropriate point on your time map. Remember: these images do not have to be distinct or vivid; they just have to be there. Then, as you actually go through the time period in question, keep reminding yourself to visualize where you are on your cognitive map. If you can train yourself to do this, you will have vastly increased your own internal resources. You will be helping yourself avoid the inconvenience of losing track of time and failing to meet your obligations. You may be able to replace feelings of frustration and failure with feelings of being clever and competent. And, you may inspire more confidence in others.

—▬—

CHAPTER 17
Method Seven
The Sense Convergence Method

———

Even for a person operating at peak efficiency, it
is a genuine challenge to respond in a coordinated
fashion to all the stimuli impinging on us.

THE SENSE CONVERGENCE METHOD IS a technique I developed while leading self-hypnosis workshops at a university years ago. This method will appear at first glance to be most odd and unusual. However, it may also be one that has great potential to help you train your own neurological system to do a better job sorting through and responding to the stimuli of daily life.

First, I am assuming that you will have learned the brief relaxation method described in Chapter 11. If not, then when these instructions ask you to do the brief relaxation method, instead simply take 4 to 6 slow, deep breaths.

Make a selection of three common tasks that you have to perform frequently in your home. These are to be tasks that require no more than five minutes to perform. In addition, select tasks that you do not really enjoy - tasks that usually make you feel uncomfortable, rushed or scattered when you perform them.

Next, make sure you have an insulated bottle with a narrow neck, such as a thermos bottle. It must be a bottle that makes a continuous change in pitch as it is filled with water from a tap (actually, the pitch of the sound rises because the column of air left in the bottle is growing shorter). Follow the following steps.

- Stand at the kitchen sink, and place the thermos bottle under the tap.
- Perform your brief relaxation exercise two times (or, take 4 to 6 slow, deep breaths).
- Close your eyes, and open the tap. Listen carefully to the sound of the bottle filling, and turn off the tap in a smooth motion so that you have turned off the water smoothly as the bottle is becoming full.
- Reduce your world to two sensations: the sound of the bottle filling and the feeling of turning off the tap.
- Empty the bottle and repeat. Perform this exercise several times, until you have achieved a smooth, enjoyable feeling of coordination between the sound of the bottle filling and the feeling of turning off the tap.
- Do your brief relaxation exercise two more times (or, take 4 to 6 slow, deep breaths).
- Perform your three tasks.

After completing your three tasks, consider what the experience has been like. I have had scores of patients perform this exercise, and their responses are varied, but almost universally positive. Some patients simply state that they performed their three tasks without much thought, and were surprised that they were done so easily. Some patients have been much more specific. They have given me accounts of doing a well-considered, efficient job on food preparation, kitchen clean-up tasks, et cetera. For instance, without consciously planning to do so, they have filled their dishwasher in a more efficient way. Or, while preparing food, they have found themselves, again without the conscious plan to do so, arranging, preparing and mixing ingredients in a more effective manner. Importantly, they report feeling more relaxed and comfortable while performing the tasks.

What is going on here? How can filling a thermos bottle make a change in a person's experience of doing tasks? Once again, let us go back to the phenomenology of ADHD. Every one of us, in all our conscious moments, encounters an array of stimuli. When we consider all the sights, sounds, objects-in-motion, aromas, plans, expectations and obligations that make up our phenomenological field, it can be a dizzying array. Furthermore, we have to make responses to that array of stimuli. Even for a person operating at peak efficiency, it is a genuine challenge to respond in a coordinated fashion to all the stimuli impinging on us. Moreover, if we are fatigued, distracted, or have ADHD-like tendencies, it is that much more difficult. When we are distracted, ineffective or inefficient, we can define this as a lack of coordination between the stimuli we are facing and our responses to those stimuli.

Recall the instructions I gave on filling the thermos bottle: "Perform this exercise several times, until you have achieved a smooth, enjoyable feeling of coordination between the sound of the bottle filling and the feeling of turning off the tap." During those moments when you were filling the thermos, you had reduced all the world's stimuli to one sound: the sound of the bottle filling. And, you had reduced all your responses to the world to one motion: turning off the tap. You were instructed to enjoy that feeling of coordination. This is why I call the technique the "sense convergence method." You are creating a convergence between a stimulus and a response - between a sound you hear and a motion you perform. For those few moments, you achieved a state of excellent coordination between the world's stimulation and your responses. If you did your tasks more efficiently, you must have brought some of that excellent coordination with you. You had changed your internal state. You had created a state of mind that was better able to manage your responses to the world. For those moments, you had successfully combatted your ADHD.

I had an experience many years ago when I was practicing in Texas. I had a client who had terrible allergy problems. He would be sniffing and snorting constantly during sessions. He was a 26-year old man who was just in the process of completing his bachelor's degree. He informed me that he had lost many years of school due to the severity of his allergies, and that his allergies were persistent and intractable. As he seemed to have some distractibility issues, I had him do the thermos bottle exercise. When he came back in, he had done the exercise, and had experienced the expected sense of improved comfort and efficiency when doing his three tasks. Then he told me that his allergies were much better.

I was stunned. To this day, I do not know for sure what was at work. Was it a coincidence? Remember: the brain controls the body. Moreover, at a basic level, what is an allergy problem? It is a lack of coordination between a stimulus (an environmental pathogen) and the body's response (inappropriately high immune response). Remember one of the ways I have been describing ADHD. It is a lack of coordination between environmental stimulation and our responses to that stimulation. Is it possible that at some level of neurological functioning, the client's experience of coordination while doing the sense convergence method began to retrain his immune system? I have no idea. However, I do believe that the sense convergence method has potential to be a powerful tool. Use it to re-train yourself to be better coordinated in your responses to the demands, obligations and other stimuli in your life.

I highly recommend not only that you practice the sense convergence method with the thermos bottle, but that you also look for other ways to apply it in your life. Let us consider some possibilities. When you are driving your car, watch the line of traffic in front of you. When you see that the cars in front are becoming bunched up, let up on the accelerator. You are creating a convergence between the distance between cars ahead of you and your application of pressure on your gas pedal. This particular use of the sense convergence method may save your life, or at least prevent an accident.

Let us consider the volume of a television or stereo. Many persons make adjustments in an abrupt manner. If they think the volume is too low, they quickly make it much higher. Then, if they have made it too high, they quickly make it much lower. They may continue in this manner, alternating between too high and too low a level of volume. An alternative would be to start by raising the volume a little, paying careful attention to your comfort level with the volume. If you have not raised it enough, raise it a little more, and so on, until you reach a good comfort level.

Adjusting our driving speed to the line of traffic in front of us and adjusting the volume level to our comfort level are actions in response to immediate feedback. But, what about longer term adjustments in more complicated circumstances? College students might adjust their study time according to the level of approval they sense from professors. Supervisors in a work situation might adjust their level of praise and encouragement according to the level of morale and productivity they see in their workers.

Let us consider an even more complicated example. Suppose you have not been on good terms with a family member due to longstanding issues. For the sake of discussion, let us call him "Jake." You may not feel that "having it out" with Jake would be helpful, and you may not feel that there is any "quick fix." However, let us assume you do value the relationship and you do not want it to remain frigid and distant forever. Perhaps there is a way of responding that would be somewhat analogous to the task of gradually raising the volume level to a comfortable level.

As the holiday season approaches, you may send Jake a card. If he does not send a card in return, and does not say "thanks" at a family gathering, you may want to hold off on your next gesture. However, if he does acknowledge your card, you may want to make another gesture, such as a phone call. Again, if his response is neutral or distant, you may wait awhile. But if he responds with even a little warmth, you may plan your next gesture, such as an invitation to join you for coffee or lunch.

At every juncture, you gauge Jake's response to your gradually increasing overtures, and you raise your gesture to the next level. This process may take days, weeks or months. The important point is that you would be gradually working toward a desired end, continually adjusting your actions to the responses you receive in return. This is a much more complicated and lengthy situation than adjusting your turning off a tap to the sound of air escaping a thermos bottle, but the concept is the same. Moreover, the more often you look for situations that are analogous in some way to the thermos bottle exercise, the more coordinated will be your overall responses to the changing world around you. When in doubt, go back to the thermos bottle exercise and look for the simple situations to which to bring the feeling of coordination.

———————

CHAPTER 18
Method Eight
The Method of Loci

———

T HE METHOD OF LOCI IS more than two thousand years old. "Loci" is the plural of the Latin word "Locus," which means "place." Therefore, this is the "Method of Places." Greek orators in ancient Athens used this method to remember the topics they wanted to address in a speech. Ever since human beings began living in cities and practicing agriculture about 6,000 years ago, each generation had copious amounts of information to pass on to the next. People had to know how to commit things to memory: stories, legends, traditions, planting times and practices. Written materials were not available. People had to develop their internal memory, whereas today we are not obliged to do so, since we have so many paper and electronic ways to store information in "external memory."

HOW DOES THE METHOD OF LOCI WORK?

First, you have to commit to memory a series of physical places. To make it as easy as possible you will want to memorize a series of places that you know well, and that either are or were part of your life. Following are a couple of examples of how a person might go about memorizing a series of places.

You may want to use the sequence of places in your home, as though you were getting up, taking care of hygiene, getting a hot beverage, getting dressed, having breakfast, leaving the house, getting into your car, and pulling out onto the road:

1. Sitting on the side of your bed before you rise
2. Your bathroom
3. The kitchen appliance where you prepare tea or coffee
4. Your closet where you select clothes for the day
5. Your breakfast table
6. The door by which you leave the house
7. Your carport or garage
8. The street, as you pull away from home.

Now let us consider a simple way in which you might put this series of eight places to use. Suppose you needed to go to the supermarket, and you needed eight items:

1. A head of lettuce
2. Three red bell peppers
3. Grapefruit
4. A dozen eggs
5. A carton of milk
6. Three cans of green beans
7. Oil and vinegar
8. Salmon filets

To use the method of loci to memorize your list, you have to make images. The method works best when the images are striking in some way.

Imagery is an interesting phenomenon in and of itself. Clinicians often assume that imagery will be visual. In fact, many use the term "visualization." For many therapeutic endeavors, it is much more powerful to create images using all the senses, particularly the big three: sight, sound and touch. We tend to vary in terms of the relative strength of our imagery skills in these three senses. Let us consider how a person might go about memorizing the grocery list shown above.

1. Imagine encountering a head of lettuce as you are about to rise. You might see a huge head of lettuce blocking your way. You could imagine rising and stepping on the head of lettuce, in which case you could emphasize the feeling of the lettuce under your foot and the crunching sound it makes as you put your weight on it.

2. Imagine going into the bathroom, and instead of the mirror there is a picture of three red bell peppers.

3. Imagine that instead of coffee or tea you are squeezing grapefruit for juice. You could imagine the feeling of squeezing the grapefruit, or the sound of the juice being squeezed out of the fruit.

4. Imagine being in your closet, reaching for shoes, and finding a carton of a dozen eggs instead.

5. Imagine sitting down to breakfast, picking up a carton of milk and finding it empty. Imagine the lightness of it, and imagine hearing your own voice saying, "How can I have breakfast with no milk?"

6. Imagine leaving your house, tripping on something, and looking back to see that you have tripped over three cans of green beans.

7. Imagine preparing to sit in the driver's seat of your car, and seeing large bottles of oil and vinegar right where you had hoped to sit.

8. Imagine trying to pull out onto the street, only to have your way blocked by a man with a pushcart. He is selling fish and holding up a huge salmon fillet.

If you had already committed those eight places to memory, and then went through the exercise of making those eight images, it is very likely you will remember all your items at the store, even without a written list.

Let us think of another example of a series of places, and another example of a series of items to remember. Here is an example of a high school student, memorizing a list of places he typically visits during a school day.

1. In the bedroom closet, selecting clothes for the day
2. In the kitchen, eating breakfast
3. At the bus stop, waiting for the school bus
4. Walking up the front steps to the school
5. At locker
6. In homeroom
7. In school auditorium.
8. In gymnasium.

Now let us imagine that our hypothetical student has to give an oral presentation on the history of science. Imagine he has to give some information about each of the following figures in the history of science:

1. Archimedes
2. Ptolemy
3. Copernicus
4. Galileo
5. Sir Isaac Newton

6. Edwin Hubble
7. Albert Einstein
8. Nils Bohr

1. You may recall that Archimedes was famous for his law of displacement. Our student may imagine a tub of water with the displaced water spilling all over the shoes in his closet.
2. The Ptolemaic System was a model of our solar system that had the Earth in the center. Our student might imagine sitting at the breakfast table watching an orange in orbit around a grape, signifying the now long-discarded notion that the Sun revolves around the Earth.
3. Copernicus was one of many astronomers who finally unseated the Ptolemaic System, but putting the Sun in its rightful place at the center of the solar system is often attributed to him. Our student might make an image of Copernicus, standing on top of a school bus, working on a model of the Solar System, physically wrenching a model of the Sun from its orbit and placing it in the center.
4. Galileo is given credit for inventing the telescope, with which he discovered the four largest moons (the Galilean moons) of Jupiter. Our student may simply imagine that as he mounts the steps to school, someone is looking at him through an enormous telescope.
5. Newton wrote Principia Mathematica Philosophae Naturalis. He is best known for his law of gravity. There is a story, probably apocryphal, of Newton being hit on the head by an apple. Our student may simply imagine being hit on the head by an apple while standing at his locker.
6. Edwin Hubble, after whom our space telescope is named, discovered that our Universe is expanding. Our student might

imagine sitting in his homeroom watching the walls and ceiling of the room expanding.

7. Albert Einstein, whose special and general theories of relativity revolutionized physics, is probably the best know of all scientists in history. Pictures of him with an unkempt mop of white hair are common. Our student may image being in the school auditorium and seeing Einstein on the stage.

8. Nils Bohr was one of many physicists who developed the quantum theory that postulates, among other things, that energy is not continuous, but exists in tiny packets, or quanta. For instance, an electron must exist at certain energy states around the nucleus of an atom; it cannot occupy an energy state in between. Our student may imagine that a shot put or discus cannot land anywhere, but appears to have to land at certain distances from the athlete.

If our hypothetical student were to make vivid images as described above, he would probably be able to move his discussion from one scientist to the next without skipping a beat.

A few last points about the method of loci:

-   Persons wishing to use this method may commit to memory two or three series of places, or as many as they want. It is, of course, best to have a particular set of places very firmly in mind before establishing another.
-   Contestants in memory championships often go through the process of erasing their images one by one when they no longer need them. Some of them report that this makes it easier for them to utilize the loci again in the future without interference from a previously used image.

- The more vivid, even outlandish, are the images a person creates, the more likely they are to be recalled.

———

CHAPTER 19
Method Nine
Do Ten Things

———

THE "DO TEN THINGS" METHOD is a good method for just about everyone and not just for persons with ADHD. We very often find ourselves procrastinating on tasks. Individuals who regard themselves as perfectionists are particularly susceptible to procrastination. Perfectionists are reluctant even to begin a task if they feel they do not have the time, resources and energy to do a perfect job.

One of the most common reasons for procrastination is that the task feels too big, complicated or formidable to us at the moment we are facing it. In many instances, the "Do Ten Things" method allows us to take what would otherwise be a formidable task and cut it down to a non-formidable, approachable size.

One very common example is straightening up a house or apartment. You probably know at least one or two persons who have difficulty keeping their house or apartment neat and uncluttered. You may even know someone who expresses frustration at times due to his or her inability to maintain a more consistently organized home. Their homes may therefore at times be a very cluttered mess. Here is an example of how the "Do Ten Things" method can help.

We are facing a really cluttered mess, and straightening it all out would seem to be a task requiring a great deal of time, effort and motivation. Instead of even considering doing the whole job, we decide to do ten things. We see yesterday's newspaper on a table. We put it in the recycle bin and say, "one." There is a jacket hanging over the arm of a sofa. We hang it up in the closet and say, "two." A pair of running shoes is on the floor. We put them in the closet and say, "three." Two coffee mugs are on a coffee table. We place them in the kitchen sink and say, "four." There is a box of cereal on the kitchen table. We put it in a pantry cupboard and say, "five." A book is on the arm of a chair. We put it on the appropriate shelf and say, six." There is a pair of pliers on the floor. We put it into the appropriate drawer or toolbox and say, "seven." A DVD sits on top of the television. We put it on its appropriate shelf and say, eight." A recently purchased package of batteries sits in the plastic bag in which we brought it home. We toss the bag or place it in the recyclables, put the batteries in the appropriate drawer and say, "nine." There is a T-shirt handing on the back of a chair. We put it in the laundry basket or hamper and say, "ten!" Then, we stop. Yes, we really do stop.

You may ask, "Isn't it possible that, having seen how much better things appear now that I have done ten things, I may experience a rush of energy and motivation? Isn't it possible I may really be 'on a roll,' and I may want to get the whole job done?"

Yes, it is very possible – even likely – that this will happen at least some of the time. However, it is vitally important that you do stop after "ten" some, if not most, of the time. Why? Because if you are using the "Do Ten Things" method as a ploy or subterfuge to maneuver yourself into doing the entire task, you will begin to avoid "ten things" just as you would avoid the entire job. Therefore, it is very important that you really do stop after ten things most of the time you use the method.

How long does it take to "Do Ten Things"?

In the example I described above, each of the tasks would be a twenty-to-thirty second task. Therefore, in that example three-to-five minutes would suffice. If some of the tasks require going up and down a flight of stairs, or taking a quick trip out to a garage or car, we may be looking at eight-to-ten minutes. This method, in the form in which I am presenting it, works best if the tasks are quick, allowing the entire ten things to be accomplished in five minutes or less.

When is it a good time to "Do Ten Things"?

- Right before going to bed.
- Before leaving the house for work or school, if you find yourself ready a few minutes ahead of time.
- While something is heating in the oven or microwave.
- During a television commercial break.
- While waiting for a return phone call.
- While waiting for a visitor to arrive.
- Before sitting down to a more involved task, such as paying bills or reading a chapter in a book.
- As a break in the middle of a more involved task.
- As soon as you walk in the door, before sitting down to relax.
- First thing in the morning, as soon as you rise.

Use your own imagination and best judgment to decide when to do ten things. You will find that, depending on the number of persons in your home, and their personal habits, if you "Do Ten Things" three times per day, your home may never approach perfection, but it will never deteriorate into a cluttered mess.

WHAT ARE SOME OTHER USES OF "DO TEN THINGS" BESIDES KEEPING A HOME UNCLUTTERED?

- Going through and dealing with accumulated mail and other papers.
- Cleaning out the trunk of a car.
- Taking out and folding clothes from the drier.
- Emptying a dish drainer or dishwasher.
- Organizing a basement or workroom.
- Pulling weeds from a garden or planting area.

IS "TEN" A MAGIC NUMBER?

No, it is not. Ten is a good number when cleaning up a house or apartment. Perhaps you would prefer the number SIX when emptying a dish drainer or folding items from a clothes drier. Make up your own rules for different situations. However, once you set a rule, stick to it unless it truly requires an adjustment. Consistency is important if a method such as this one is to work for you.

———

CHAPTER 20
Method Ten
Soliloquy

———

MY REAL NAME FOR THIS method is "keeping up a running commentary." In drama, a soliloquy is a speech by actors, ostensibly to themselves, but actually for the benefit of the audience. In this case, keeping up a running commentary is really for your own benefit.

When individuals with ADHD or ADHD-like issues describe their frustrations, they frequently complain of episodes such as the following:

- I often drive right by my exit on the highway.
- I sometimes leave water running in a sink or bathtub, go to do something else, forget the running water, and overflow the sink or tub.
- I sometimes leave something on the stove or in the oven and forget it is there.

One remedy is to keep up a running commentary – a soliloquy, if you will. If you are alone, you may actually speak aloud to yourself. If you are with others, an internal commentary will prevent you from appearing odd or eccentric. For instance, if you are driving on Route 95 north to come to my office, you may begin around exit 20 by telling yourself, "Four more exits to go to the Branch Avenue exit." A moment later, you may tell yourself, "I'm going to see Dr. Slavit, so I have to take exit 24." Another moment later you may say, "Yep. I'll get into the right lane and be ready to take exit 24."

It is very important that you change the wording of what you say to yourself. The reason for this is that otherwise you will habituate to the words, the same way you habituate to the sound of a fan or air conditioner. Thus, if you simply keep saying, "Take exit 24. Take exit 24. Take exit 24," the words will lose their meaning. They will no longer register in your mind as a new stimulus for you to understand, and you may drive right by exit 24 while repeating the same warning to yourself.

Another technique you may use while using a running commentary is to change the emphasis you place on different words. Thus, you may tell yourself:

- *I* will return to the sink and shut off the running water.
- I *WILL* return to the sink and shut off the running water.
- I will *RETURN* to the sink and shut off the running water.
- I will return to *THE* sink and shut off the running water.
- I will return to the *SINK* and shut off the running water.
- I will return to the sink and turn *OFF* the running water.
- I will return to the sink and turn off the running *WATER*.

Anything that keeps the stimulus novel, whether a change in the wording or a change in the emphasis, will help prevent you from habituating to the stimulus and making the error you are trying to avoid.

Keeping a running commentary may seem peculiar. It is not the first method of choice for most daily tasks and activities. However, in situations such as the ones described – running water in a tub, a pot on the stove, or remembering to take the correct exit off the highway – it may prove helpful to avoid significant inconvenience.

———

CHAPTER 21
Method Eleven
The 60/40 Principle

———

THE 60/40 PRINCIPLE IS PROBABLY the loosest and least well defined of the twenty methods described. Nevertheless, it is a very important organizing principle for effective living. First, I will describe an hypothetical situation that gives an idea of the issue, and I will then illustrate the 60/40 principle.

Let us assume you have a child who is playing little league baseball, and you have to arrive at the game before it ends to bring him/her home. Let us also assume that the recreational facility at which the games are played contains ten ball fields. You can imagine that it might take you a great deal of time and energy to locate your child. Perhaps your child's team uniform is similar to others, and not easy to spot. In addition, your child may be in the dugout or at a water cooler at the moment you scan that field to locate him/her. You can easily imagine that locating your child among ten ball fields could end up being a lengthy and frustrating process.

Now imagine a slightly different scenario. Imagine that the little league officials have informed you that teams in your child's division will be playing their games on fields one through four. This makes your task much easier, and the lengthy, frustrating experience described in the previous example would be very unlikely.

The 60/40 principle can be applied very specifically in some situations, and as a loose, organizing principle in others. It offers some distinct advantages that will be explained.

EXAMPLE ONE: THE REFRIGERATOR

Yes, life often revolves around the kitchen, and the refrigerator is an important center of activity. How well organized does a refrigerator have to be for its use to be reasonably efficient? Does there have to be either A) a specific place for every single item that might be stored there? Alternatively, B) can we live efficiently in our kitchen by just putting things into the refrigerator wherever we find space at that moment?

I believe that the answer to both the above questions is a solid "No." Having a specific place for every single item would be impractical, time-consuming, and unnecessary. In fact, it would be so time consuming and arduous that attempting method "A" would inevitably lead to method "B." Why? For one thing, while there are some items you will typically have on hand, there are probably scores of other items that are on hand occasionally or seldom, and having a system that would include a place for them would be a waste of your time. For another thing, having a specific place for every item in your refrigerator would be an exercise in compulsive behavior – not an exercise in effective living.

Why do I say that attempting method "A" would inevitably lead to method "B"? And what are the broader implications for combatting ADHD and for effective living? If you tried to have a specific place for every item that you might ever have in your fridge, you would be spending a great deal of time devising a rulebook for that system. You would also spend a great deal of time and effort referring to your rulebook, and rearranging items to meet criteria. This activity would be so time consuming that it would inevitably lose out in competition with other obligations. You would then abandon the system in frustration and, with no back-up system in place, your fridge would quickly decay to total chaos. You would then have the time-wasting activities of searching for items you need. Stored items would "go bad" because they would be shoved behind other items and be ignored. Frustration and a sense of failure would ensue. And, if this scenario were played out in other areas of your life in addition to your refrigerator, you would very likely develop low self esteem and a feeling that your life will inevitably be disorganized, chaotic and unsatisfying. You would, in fact, conclude that you are and will forever be a disorganized, incompetent person.

So, how would the 60/40 principle apply? I will illustrate this by first naming ten items you might possibly find in someone's fridge.

1. Orange juice
2. Soy milk
3. Cottage cheese
4. Eggs
5. Mayonnaise
6. Catsup
7. Blueberries
8. Olives
9. Tomorrow's lunch sandwich
10. Tonight's dinner leftovers

Now let us suppose that you have designated the left and middle of the tall shelf for orange juice and soy milk. Suppose there is a medium height shelf on which you always keep your cottage cheese. Eggs are always kept on the low shelf, and mayonnaise and catsup are always kept on the refrigerator door. Where should items 7 through 10 go? Who cares? Wherever they are, they will be easy to spot, because you will only have forty percent of the total space to search for them. Remember the baseball field analogy. You can easily find your child if you can ignore six fields and only have to locate him among four fields.

Example Two: A Day of Errands

Now let us assume that you have a day ahead of you in which there are ten errands and activities that you hope to accomplish. Once again, I have chosen the number ten since it can be easily divided into a 60/40 split. Ten hypothetical errands and activities are as follows:

1. Work out at the fitness Center
2. Buy stamps at the post office
3. Pick up groceries at the supermarket
4. Phone in a prescription & pick it up later
5. Put fuel in the car
6. Write a birthday card for Uncle Bob
7. Start packing for next weeks' vacation trip
8. Read a travel brochure about your vacation destination
9. Call Mom
10. marinate chicken for tonight's supper

Let us suppose you attempt method "A". You write out the following schedule:

8:00	–	8:30	phone in prescription
8:30	–	10:00	work out at fitness center
10:00	–	10:30	buy stamps at post office
10:30	–	11:15	pick up groceries at market
11:15	–	11:30	put fuel in car
11:30	–	11:45	write birthday card for Uncle

11:45	–	1:00	lunch
1:00	–	2:30	pack for next week vacation
2:30	–	4:00	read travel brochure about travel destination
4:00	–	4:30	call Mom
4:30	–	5:00	pick up prescription
5:00	–	5:30	marinate chicken for tonight's supper

Do you believe you would be happy or successful trying to follow such a schedule? I think it should be obvious that such a schedule would result in failure. Any number of events could happen that would cause such a schedule to fail, such as a phone call or visit from a friend or relative. Moreover, even if, against all odds, you did manage on an occasion to follow such a schedule, it is more likely you would feel "hemmed in" and overly structured than that you would feel relaxed, happy and efficient.

Let us suppose, then, that you try method "B". You are aware of the ten errands and activities, and, without any planning or scheduling at all, you just tell yourself, "There are a lot of hours in the day. I'll just see how it goes." Do you think you will accomplish all ten? Do you think it will be a comfortable day? Do you think the day will end with you having a sense of competence or mastery? The answer to all three questions is, "It is very unlikely."

How would we approach such a list of errands and activities using the 60/40 principle? First, let us look for a few organizing ideas. Phoning in the prescription has to be done early in the day so that it can be picked up later. Obviously, groceries must be purchased before the chicken can be marinated. Perhaps you do not have good concentration for reading later in the day, so reading the travel brochure has to be done early. Perhaps you prefer a fitness center workout to be early in the day when the fitness center is less crowded. Lastly, due to the preference for a gym workout early, and the need to pick up a prescription later, there will have to be at least two trips from the house.

Given these organizing ideas and the 60/40 principle, let us look at the following agenda:

- early morning call in prescription
- mid morning leave home, work out at fitness center and, on the way home, pick up groceries
- late morning read travel brochure
- afternoon go out, buy stamps, fuel car, and pick up prescription

But, wait? What about Uncle Bob's birthday card, calling Mom, packing, and marinating the chicken? When we they be done? Who cares? You can fit them in among the other activities when you feel like it. Six of your ten agenda items are scheduled, and the other four can be taken care of without excessive planning. You can be efficient, effective and successful without having a rigid, oppressive schedule.

ARE THE NUMBERS "60/40" IMPORTANT?

No, they are not. In fact, there are instances in which you may want to revise them. Let us take an example regarding health and nutrition. I know a nurse practitioner who treats Lyme Disease using a number of methods, including some holistic approaches. She favors a healthful regimen of natural foods and supplements. She promotes what she calls "the 80/20 rule." She tells her patients that if they adhere to a healthy regimen eighty percent of the time, they do not have to be overly concerned about twenty percent indulgences.

Let us assume that there is a history of heart disease in your family and your physician advises you to adhere to a "heart healthy diet." Do you believe that 60/40 is a good principle in this instance? Do you think it is wise to stray from a healthy eating regimen forty percent of the time? Alternatively, are the possible consequences of forty percent indulgent eating too much of a risk? I suspect that the consequences are too dire for most people to accept. On the other hand, do you want to strive for 100/0? Do you want to live without ever having an ice cream cone on a summer afternoon? Do you want to live without ever having a hamburger or hot dog at a summer cookout? Do you want to refuse to ever have a slice of cake at someone's birthday party? I suspect that 100/0 is unattainable and that 80/20 would be a more reasonable principle.

Let us take another example. Suppose you have purchased a kayak, paddle and life jacket. You have been taking your kayak to some pond, lake or bay, and have been going out on the water. Suppose that without any instruction or coaching you have taught yourself a paddling style. Your style allows you to go with sufficient speed and to maneuver your kayak. You are able to enjoy the beauty of nature, to get moderate exercise, and to return with no discomfort or strained muscles. Then, some hotshot kayaking expert observes you and tells you he can teach you ten ways to improve your stroke. He tells you he can show you how to improve your grip of the paddle, to reach forward to the correct degree, to utilize your body's core appropriately, et cetera. Is there a recommended principle in this instance?

Perhaps you are happy with your current level of kayaking skill. It meets your need to get out into nature and to get moderate exercise. Perhaps you have been dedicating yourself to improving many aspects of your life. Maybe you want kayaking to be a relaxed and casual activity with no performance standards. Perhaps 0/100 is an acceptable principle for you in this instance. In other words, perhaps you are happy with your kayaking activities just as they are and you feel no need at all to increase your efficiency at this pastime.

Let us take another example of a situation in which 60/40 might not be desirable: driving a car. Let us suppose you are taught the following rules of safe driving:

1. Stop at all red lights.
2. Stop at all stop signs.
3. At a stop sign, look left, right and then left before proceeding.
4. Drive at or under the speed limit.
5. Drive below the speed limit when the road is wet.
6. Stay a safe distance behind the vehicle in front of you.
7. Always signal your turns.
8. Always signal your lane changes.
9. Stop driving and rest if you feel sleepy.
10. Do not send text messages while driving.

Do you think the 60/40 principle is sufficient? If so, to which four of the ten risks do you want to subject yourself, your passengers, and other drivers? I think it should be clear that 100/0 is the appropriate principle to follow for driving safety.

WHAT ARE THE BASIC MESSAGES OF THE 60/40 PRINCIPLE?

- Life is a happier, more satisfying affair when we live with some degree of effectiveness, efficiency and productivity.
- It is therefore worthwhile to engage in at least moderate striving to do well.
- Every human being has some degree of ADHD, or ADHD-like issues.
- Striving for perfection is unwise, as it cannot be attained. If we strive for perfection, we will not attain it. We will then feel discouraged, which will reduce our self-esteem, and in turn reduce our motivation.

- The 60/40 principle is intended to be an organizing concept around which we can set and work toward goals.
- Whether it is your refrigerator, your schedule for a day, the top of your desk or the trunk of your car, if you let it decay into a cluttered mess, you will experience inconvenience and frustration. If you organize a significant portion of it . . . oh, say . . . sixty percent . . . the rest of it will become much more manageable without a tiresome, obsessive effort.
- As to perfection: *you cannot do this. As to the 60/40 principle: you can do this.*

———

CHAPTER 22
Method Twelve
The Reverse Agenda

—■—

PRODUCTIVITY AND EFFICIENCY ARE WORTHWHILE goals to which many of us subscribe. Many persons use the method of written agendas to keep track of the tasks and obligations facing them. This can serve the purpose of preventing an important task or obligation from being left uncompleted. In addition, giving ourselves a bold checkmark – preferably with a flourish – can be reinforcing when we have completed a task from our list.

However, there are potential risks associated with writing out our tasks and obligations in advance. This may be particularly true for persons with ADHD. Remember what I have been saying in different ways about the phenomenological experience of persons with ADHD. When the stimuli facing them appear complicated, confusing or formidable, they are subject to either disorganized responses or escapism. Whether we have ADHD or not, we may very well look at an agenda list and find it daunting, or even overwhelming. This will tend to reduce our motivation to begin. In addition, if the agenda is too long for completion in a day, we may feel the need to stay task oriented at the expense of relaxation, recreation or our social lives.

My suggested remedy is to reverse the process. When you are aware of tasks and obligations, set out a sheet of paper and simply put the day and date at the top. Go ahead and perform a task, preferably starting with an easy task. Then go to your reverse agenda sheet and list the task, along with a checkmark. Go do another task, and again write it down after completion. Proceed in this manner, writing down tasks *only when they have been completed*. As your list grows, so will grow your sense of accomplishment, and with it your motivation to continue. In addition, you will be focusing primarily on what you have done, rather than on what is left undone.

You may even have a number in mind — a number of tasks that to you represent a reasonable degree of productivity. Perhaps you like the number 10 and, after you have completed ten tasks, you feel that you have been responsible and productive and allow yourself to turn to restorative activities such as recreation, relaxation or social activity.

Productivity, efficiency and task completion are worthy goals, and are part of living a satisfying, meaningful life. But when pursuing these goals feels like self-oppression, we may have forgotten the other goal of living a satisfying, happy life.

In the words from the poem Desiderata, by Max Ehrmann:

Beyond a wholesome discipline, be gentle with yourself.
You are a child of the Universe, no less than the trees and the stars.
You have a right to be here.

—■—

CHAPTER 23
Method Thirteen
Break it Down

—■—

I N THE PREVIOUS CHAPTER, I introduced you to the "Reverse Agenda," a method designed to help you to avoid the tyranny of a formidable agenda. By reversing the agenda process and writing down tasks **after** you have accomplished them, you will avoid procrastination and will experience increased motivation and energy as your list of completed tasks grows.

However, there could be a problem if you follow the reverse agenda method exclusively. Writing down your completed tasks will give you a sense of diligence and competence. However, it is possible that you will gain a false sense of security. You may feel that, having been task oriented and diligent, you have fulfilled your responsibilities. This could especially be true if you had set a goal of a certain number of tasks and have attained that number. Can you see the possible problem?

If you had a particularly difficult or lengthy task ahead of you, it is possible that you may avoid that task completely. Less formidable tasks may be seen as an easy but legitimate escape from the difficult task. When I was in graduate school, many times I heard other students say that their apartments had never been neater and cleaner than when exams were coming. This was because they were allowing themselves to feel conscientious by cleaning their apartments. However, they were avoiding the more formidable task of studying for exams. Similarly, you may avoid a difficult task and not feel a sense of unease about it, as you have in fact been productive and responsible. However, there are times when you need to perform a difficult, lengthy or otherwise formidable task in order to avoid inconvenient consequences.

The solution to this problem is to break the tough task down into smaller, doable steps. As an example, suppose you are taking an academic course and have a research paper to write. When you think of all that you must do to complete that task, it may appear in your consciousness as a jumble of individual tasks. You are thinking about going to the library to find books and articles. You are thinking about narrowing down a more general assignment to a specific area of focus. You are thinking about reading some articles, or chapters of books, and taking notes. You are thinking about sorting through your notes to arrange them in a coherent order. You are thinking about writing a first draft. You are thinking about reading your first draft, identifying areas of weakness and going back to source materials to seek further information. You are thinking about adding the new material to the weak parts of your work. You are thinking about writing a final draft. You are thinking about proofreading your final draft and making any needed corrections. All of these tasks may be swirling around in your mind in a dizzying fashion, creating a sense that the task is formidable, and therefore creating a desire to escape.

It will be important for you to teach yourself that seemingly complex and difficult tasks can be broken down into small steps that are doable. You do not have to experience complex tasks as formidable. Think about the very first step listed above: Go to the library to find books and articles. You may need to focus on that one step, and to momentarily put thoughts of later steps out of your mind. Only after going to the library and acquiring your books and articles will it be helpful for you to think about the next step: reading some articles, or chapters of books, and taking notes. If you are using the reverse agenda method, write down each step you have accomplished and give yourself a checkmark. If you are starting your research paper ahead of time, one step per day may be sufficient. Moreover, if you do take one step per day, you will not feel the task is formidable, and you will not have the strong desire to escape the project.

Research papers are obviously not the only tasks that may initially appear to be complex and difficult. Tax returns, packing for a vacation, cleaning a house or apartment, re-arranging a basement, clearing off a desk and filing important documents, folding and storing the clothes from a clothes drier, doing a spring clean up of a lawn and garden, or cleaning up after Thanksgiving dinner can all qualify.

Let us look at a second example: cleaning up after a large holiday dinner. Many of us have had the following experience. We have been invited to a holiday dinner such as Thanksgiving dinner. Having enjoyed our host's hospitality, we decide to reciprocate by cleaning up. We march into the kitchen, full of resolve, only to be confronted with a very big mess. The sink is full of pots and pans. The leftover turkey and many other foods are on the kitchen table, along with stacks of dishes, utensils, used napkins, et cetera. You look from one side of the kitchen to the other and back again. You try to decide where to begin, but you feel so overwhelmed by the complexity of the task that you walk out of the kitchen, saying, "I think I will get another piece of pie."

How can we break such a complex task down into achievable steps? First we look for some organizing principle (at this point, any organizing principle will suffice). A sense of curiosity about what that organizing principle may be, and the first step it suggests, will be helpful. A good one: make the sink usable. Therefore, we find some newspaper and put several pieces on the floor. We get the pots and pans out of the sink, and place them on the newspaper. There! We have en empty, usable sink.

Then we get the biggest pot, rinse it out, fill it halfway with hot soapy water, and put it back on the floor. We then look around for as many forks, knives, spoons and other utensils as we can find and dump them into the pot with the hot, soapy water. We have cleared out the sink, so there is enough room under the faucet to wash things. So, one at a time, we pick up the pots and pans, wash and dry them, and put them away. Things are no longer looking quite so grim.

Our eyes go to the kitchen table, which is covered with food left-overs, as well as stacks of plates, with some utensils and uneaten food between them. What a mess! We may as well make a start. We find a garbage bucket. One at a time, we take the plates, scrape leftover food and napkins into the garbage bucket, place any utensils that were hiding between plates in our pot of hot, soapy water, and stack the plates in the sink. If there is a dishwasher, we rinse the plates and put them in. If not, we wash them and place them in the dish drainer. We are really seeing our progress now. Then we find our host, ask how s/he wants leftovers stored, and begin the task of putting leftovers into containers. I think the point has been illustrated, and we do not have to describe the remaining details.

We have an idea how to handle it if we are confronted with a complicated task that looks difficult to us. First, we look for any organizing principle that will allow us to take the first step. In the case of the research paper, the first step was obvious: get the books and articles. In the case of the messy kitchen, it was not quite so obvious. However, on some reflection, the sink had to be cleared to make other tasks possible. So, getting the pots and pans out of the sink and onto the newspapers was a good step. After the first step, the next step becomes easier to approach.

I hope I have convinced you that breaking complicated, seemingly formidable tasks into achievable steps is a great way to start. In addition, I hope that the idea of looking for some organizing principle will help you to look at the complicated task with as much curiosity as fear. Life will be full of tasks that will appear to us to be unachievable. The more troubled we are with ADHD or ADHD-like issues, the more often we will feel the need to escape the task. Use the brief relaxation method (method one) to reduce your arousal level and clear your mind. Be curious about the organizing principle that will help you identify the first achievable step. Begin with that first step, and enjoy the feeling of confidence that will grow as you proceed.

CHAPTER 24
Method Fourteen
Simplify: Less is More

———

MOST OF THE METHODS I am promoting in this book are ways of strengthening your inner resources rather than methods of manipulating your environment. In this chapter, however, I am suggesting a method that involves both your inner and outer worlds. You interact with your environment in such a way that you affect your environment, and your environment in turn affects you. Many persons with ADHD have informed me that they need a simple, uncluttered setting in order to feel comfortable. Of course, this is true of many individuals and not just persons with ADHD. Whether or not you truly have ADHD, the "less is more principle" can be helpful.

The following illustration is as figurative as it is literal. So, take the specifics with a grain of salt, and look for the underlying principle. Let us assume that you have a moderate sized drawer in your kitchen. In it, you have the following items:

One.   can opener
Two.   spatula
Three.   whisk
Four.   wooden spoon

Five.	carrot peeler
Six.	garlic press
Seven.	grater
Eight.	pancake turner
Nine.	tea strainer
Ten.	serving spoon

As long as you limit yourself to ten items in the drawer, you can open the drawer, visually scan the ten items, reach the one you need, and extract it from the drawer with no difficulty. You have ten usable items. Then you acquire a bottle opener and, seeing no other place for it, you put it in the drawer. Now, the drawer is a little too full. The bottle opener gets in the way of the serving spoon, and you have only nine usable items. Then, someone gives you an egg slicer, and you add it to the drawer. The egg slicer gets in the way of the tea strainer, and you now have only eight usable items. Then you acquire a meat thermometer, and into the drawer it goes. The meat thermometer gets in the way of the pancake turner, and you now have only seven usable items. And so it goes. When the drawer has twenty items, they are so bunched in together that it appears to be a tangled mess and you have difficulty visually identifying what you want. Furthermore, even if you do find your item, you have difficulty extracting it from the drawer without pulling two other items out with it and having them fall on the floor. Finally, the twenty-item drawer has become so difficult to handle that it remains forever closed. Now you have zero usable items. Most people can identify in some way with this scenario. This concept may be true for your clothes closet, a file drawer, the trunk of your car, your car's glove compartment, the top of your workbench, et cetera.

If you want to go through your life without the distraction, disorganization, anxiety and inconvenience that ADHD can produce, you need to interact with your environment in smooth and well-coordinated ways. Remember the sense convergence method I described as method seven.

We want to achieve a smooth, coordinated relationship between the demands of our environment and our responses to it. The "less is more" concept can help you to achieve this in a practical, strategic way in your home and work environments.

———

CHAPTER 25
Method Fifteen
The Gentle Eye Sweep

———

O UR EYES ARE ESSENTIALLY AN extension of the frontal lobe of our brain. Eyes and brain are very intimately connected. That eye movements are significant has been widely recognized, as evidenced by therapy methods that have been in use in recent decades. Neurolinguistic Programming is a therapy method that first became popular in the 1970's and 1980's. In this method, practitioners watch their clients' eye movements carefully as their clients access visual, auditory and kinesthetic images and memories. Another popular therapy method in recent years has been Eye Movement Desensitization, which is typically used to help patients overcome the effects of past trauma. In EMDR, patients move their eyes back and forth to cause the left and right hemispheres of the brain to communicate repeatedly across the corpus callosum. Although Neurolinguistic Programming and EMDR are quite different as methods, they do have a similarity. They are based in part on the concept that what happens with our eyes has a profound impact on our brains.

I first developed the gentle eye sweep method while working with patients with panic disorder. Persons suffering from panic typically have a difficult time in certain situations, such as movie theatres, crowded restaurants, the highway and supermarkets. After a while, it became clear to me that my patients' problems in supermarkets typically began in the store aisles, long before they may have been stuck in a line at the cashier.

Imagine that you are in the cereal aisle of a supermarket, searching for your favorite brand of toasted oats. There is a sea of cereal boxes in front of you, in three rows, stretching far to your left and right. You are hoping to find your desired brand quickly, so you essentially play your luck. You look at the top shelf to your right. No luck there. You then let your eyes dart back down and to your left. Same result. You continue in this manner, with your eyes darting back and forth until you finally find your brand. By this time, you are very likely feeling somewhat tense and disorganized. If you are a panic sufferer, you may be starting to have symptoms of a panic attack. By causing your eyes to dart about like a ball in a pinball machine, you have caused unnecessary and disorganized activity in your brain.

First, allowing your eyes to dart back and forth is a strategy based on a false premise. You are hoping that by looking about randomly you will find your brand in less than an average time. However, is it not just as likely that you will find your target in more than the average time? You have been pursuing a strategy that is illogical and ineffective in the market. However, even more importantly, you have essentially been training yourself in general to behave in a scattered, disorganized manner. You are causing or reinforcing ADHD or ADHD-like symptoms. Remember one of my main premises in this book: *ADHD is not just something you are; it is something you do.*

The alternative is the gentle eye sweep method. Begin by looking at the top shelf on your far left. Now, sweep your eyes from left to right, at a moderate pace, keeping your eyes on the top shelf. When you have reached the far right, if you have not found your favorite toasted oats, drop your eyes to the middle shelf and sweep from right to left at a moderate pace. Once again, if you have not found your oats, drop your eyes to the bottom shelf and sweep your eyes back to the right. You may find your target early in the process, or late in the process. Over the course of shopping for many items, on average you will spend the same amount of time as you would have by playing your luck with the eye dart method. However, your brain will be more quiescent. You will feel more calm and relaxed, and you will feel clever. Moreover, very importantly, you will have trained yourself to perceive, think and behave in a way that will serve you well in ways that you have not yet even imagined. You will have combatted ADHD using your own inner resources.

CHAPTER 26
Method Sixteen
The Sensory Focus Method

———

W E HAVE ALREADY ADDRESSED THE need to relax, both with a full fifteen-minute method and with the brief twenty-second method. The sensory focus method is a very simple technique to draw our minds away from chaos and complication and to restore a more relaxed state. This is not a way to achieve a deep physical relaxation, but rather a way to quiet the mind sufficiently to serve as a platform from which to launch organized, efficient thoughts and behavior.

What I call "sensory focus" is similar to methods that other practitioners call "centering" or "mindfulness." The technique is simple. Draw your attention, in turn, to everything you can see, hear, feel, and smell or taste. For the method to be effective, the person using it needs to become aware of many aspects of the experience of each sensory modality. I will illustrate with two examples – an outdoor and an indoor example.

Imagine that you are walking along a trail through the woods on a cool, autumn day. As you walk along you become aware that you are not truly noticing or enjoying your experience of being in the woods. Instead, your mind is jumping around to various situations and obligations that you face in your life. You do not want to be thinking about those matters. You are on a trail, cannot attend to your obligations at this moment, and wish to simply enjoy being in the woods. You cannot succeed in pushing the unwanted thoughts out of your mind. However, you can leave those thoughts behind by drawing your attention to your senses.

First, see what you can see. Notice the colors that are present. Pay attention to whether there are bright, vibrant colors, or subdued colors. As it is autumn and leaves are changing color, you can see some bright, vibrant orange and gold. There is also the deep green of some evergreen trees. You can also see some more subdued browns and tans. The sky is a bright blue, with a few wispy, white clouds. There are leaves overhead, and you can see patches of sky between the leaves. The sun is partially blocked by leaves, and so the trail in front of you is dappled and spotted with sunlight and shade. Looking into the woods to either side, you can see the brown trunks of the trees. There are many pine needles on the path, some of which are still green, and many of which have turned a rusty, reddish brown.

Next, hear what you can hear. Notice if there are any loud sounds or soft sounds, and any sharp sounds or any mellow sounds. Notice the sounds coming from far away and those coming from nearby. There is a moderate breeze blowing and, as it is autumn, the sound of the leaves is mostly a crisp, rustling sound. That sound comes from nearby and is a rather sharp sound. The more distant sound of the breeze in the tree tops combines to make a characteristic distant whispery sound. There may be the occasional sound of birds. Notice whether the bird sounds are more like a singing, chirping, cooing or warbling. There may be an occasional rustling sound as a squirrel, chipmunk or other animal scurries in the undergrowth. And, every now and then you may hear the gentle, muted thud of a pine cone dropping to the ground.

Next, feel what you can feel. Notice any feelings of warmth or coolness. Notice any smooth or rough textures. Notice your body position, and be aware of any sensation of motion. You may feel the coolness of the autumn breeze against your face, and a sensation of warmth in your chest due to the exertion of hiking. You may reach out and stroke the bark of a tree, noticing that the texture is rough. You may see a smooth stone, pick it up, and feel its smooth texture. You may focus on the feeling of the softness of the bed of pine needles under foot, and the sensation of gently, rhythmically strolling along.

Last, you may notice the aromas that are present. Notice if they are sweet or pungent. There may be an earthy aroma. And, you may notice the aroma of pine.

By this time you have focused your attention on all the various details of what you can see, hear, feel and smell. If you have done so effectively, it is likely that the thoughts you were having prior to your sensory focus have disappeared. Quite literally, you have come to your senses.

You will not always be outdoors in a natural environment. In fact, more often than not you will have to use the method in a less evocative place. However, there are always stimuli for your senses of sight, sound, touch and aroma. Imagine that you are in a doctor's waiting room. Your mind is racing on a number of topics, including whether you are due to have your arm punctured with a flu shot. Your thoughts are making you uncomfortable. You cannot succeed in pushing the unwanted thoughts out of your mind. However, you can leave those thoughts behind by drawing your attention to your senses.

First, let us imagine what you might see. Notice the colors that are present. Pay attention to whether there are bright, vibrant colors, or subdued colors. The walls are a nice, pale blue color, and the carpet has a mottling of shades of grey, with a few flecks of gold. There are some art prints on the walls. One in particular is a pastoral scene of a weathered, grey barn with a corral nearby and some horses in the corral. The horses are brown with black tails and manes. The waiting room has a window on one side. Sunlight is coming in, and casts a shadow of on the floor of the window trim.

Next, hear what you can hear. Notice if there are any loud sounds or soft sounds, and notice any sharp sounds or any mellow sounds. Be aware of the sound coming from farthest away and that coming from nearest by. The air conditioning is on, and you can hear the faint, whirring hum of the fan. That is a soft and mellow sound. From outside on the road you can occasionally hear the rumbling sound of a truck on the road. That is the most distant sound you can hear. A mother and child come in the door and, as the door closes, you can hear the clicking of the latch. Though soft, it is a sharp sound. The mother takes off her child's nylon jacket, and you can hear the soft rustling of the nylon.

Next, imagine what you might feel. Notice any feelings of warmth or coolness, and any smooth or rough textures. Notice your body position, and be aware of any sensation of motion. The air temperature is slightly cool, as the air conditioning is on. You are seated on a chair with a soft, coarse fabric. You stroke the seat and feel that texture, and then move your hand to the arm of the chair, which is a smooth, polished wood. Your right leg may be crossed over your left knee, and you can feel the gentle torqueing feeling in your right knee. You move your right foot back to the floor and are aware of the sensation of having both feet flat on the floor.

Last, you may notice the aromas that are present. Notice if they are sweet or pungent. There may be a faint aroma of furniture polish.

By this time, you have focused your attention on all the various details of what you can see, hear, feel and smell. If you have done so effectively, it is likely that the thoughts you were having prior to your sensory focus have disappeared. Quite literally, you have come to your senses.

The sensory focus method can help you to quiet your mind when you have too many thoughts, when your thoughts feel as though they are racing, or when your thoughts feel like a jumble. You will need to practice the method, and train yourself to focus on all the aspects of each sense.

The following is a list of some of the aspects of each sense that you may want to train yourself to notice:

Sight:
*** What colors are present? Are they bright, vibrant colors, or subdued colors?
*** Where is the light coming from? Notice any shadows that are cast.
*** What shapes can you see? Are there any curved, rounded shapes? Are there any sharp or angular shapes?

Sound:
*** Identify any loud or soft sounds.
*** Notice if sounds are sharp or mellow.
*** Identify the sound coming from farthest away.
*** Identify the nearest sound.

Feelings:
*** Be aware of any feelings of warmth or coolness.
*** Identify textures. Are there any rough textures or any smooth textures?
*** What is your body position? What sensations are present due to your body position?
*** Do you have any sensation of motion?

Aroma:

*** Notice if aromas are sweet or pungent.

*** Notice if aromas are strong or subtle.

If you will practice your ability to identify as many aspects of your sensations of sight, hearing, touch, and smell as possible, you will be developing a valuable tool. When your thoughts seem too fast, too jumbled or irrelevant to your situation, you will be able to escape them and to get relief by coming to your senses.

———

CHAPTER 27

Method Seventeen
Planning Effective Itineraries

—■—

AN ITINERARY IS A SCHEDULE of places to visit and the times to be there. The word itinerary is typically used to describe recreational or work-related travel. However, it can also be used to describe an agenda for a day. It is this latter use of the word "itinerary" that I will discuss.

HOW STRUCTURED IS "TOO STRUCTURED"?

Before I get into the challenging task of describing how to plan an effective itinerary, I would like to address the philosophical issue of living in a highly structured, time-sensitive society. I will begin with an illustration of a very different time philosophy. Years ago, I had a close friend named Rob, who led the support team on a high altitude physiological study at 17,000 feet altitude on Mount Logan in the Yukon. Rob became friendly with a member of the team. We will call him "Pete" because I do not recall his name. Pete lived in Alaska, and invited Rob to come up some time to join him for salmon fishing. Rob agreed, and asked when he should come. When Rob recounted this conversation to me, he quoted Pete, and I will repeat it as closely as I can recall. Pete said, "Rob, you don't understand how we live up here. I cannot tell you that I will go salmon fishing this week or next. I will be aware of the weather and the pace of the thaw, and one day I will wake up and decide to go salmon fishing."

Pete probably lived with no timepieces. He probably lived by the sunrise and sunset. Those of us who, in order to survive and make a living in our urbanized, industrialized, digitized society, may think about Pete's lifestyle with a sense of longing. We may feel it would be relaxing and refreshing to be free of the time schedules and time constraints with which we live. And perhaps it would be refreshing . . . for a while. However, consider the car you drive, or the bus or train you use. Metal ores had to be mined, smelted and made into steel, copper and chrome in order for our vehicles to be built. Those processes were accomplished on a time schedule. Materials had to be delivered to factories and machined into parts on a time schedule. Assembly lines had to run on a time schedule. There are undoubtedly thousands of illustrations of how the development of our housing, clothing, food, medicines, transportation and communication devices required closer and closer time schedules as the paraphernalia of our lives became more sophisticated and precise.

There are still some niches in our society in which an individual may decide what to do, and when to do it, with a minimum of time constraints. Successful freelance artists would fit into that category. To a certain extent, commercial fishermen and forest rangers may meet that criterion. However, for most of us, failure to adhere to time schedules has negative consequences. You may question whether this is good for the human psyche. Remember that the industrial revolution occurred in mid eighteenth century. Thus, we are only about thirteen generations removed from a completely rural, agrarian society. A rural, agrarian way of life would have been far less time-structured than most of us experience today. Moreover, we are only four hundred generations removed from ancestors who had not yet developed agriculture and cities. Our species did not evolve in an environment requiring the continual awareness of time and the adherence to schedules that are requirements for most of us today. Thus, I suspect that meeting present day demands is a challenge to our psyche.

If we cannot develop a lifestyle relatively free of schedules and time demands, the alternative is to develop our ability to meet the challenges. Failure to meet time demands is likely to result in failed enterprise, disapproval by others, and disappointment in ourselves. The method of itineraries may seem detailed and persnickety. However, what if the alternative is failure, disapproval and reduced self-esteem? Therefore, even if it seems detailed and persnickety, developing effective itineraries may beat the alternative.

MAKING THE BEST OF THE NEED FOR AN ITINERARY

Most of us have lives that are somewhat complex in terms of our obligations, expectations, plans and commitments. If you have ADHD or ADHD-like issues, it may be a challenge for you to think through your obligations in a systematic way and to make effective plans to meet your obligations. As you may recall from the chapter on cognitive mapping, persons with ADHD often have a limited ability to make a cognitive map of time. Many individuals, whether they have ADHD or not, often have difficulty effectively planning a day's activities. They may try to cram in too many errands, which can lead to lateness or anxiety, or both. They may plan too few tasks, and feel that they have wasted valuable time.

I will give a hypothetical example of itinerary planning. The example I have drawn up is rather detailed. Keep in mind that much simpler itineraries may be sufficient for many of our endeavors. We will call our protagonist "Hal." We will assume that there is an end point – a place to be at a specified time at the conclusion of all other errands or activities. Let us assume that the end point is that tomorrow Hal wants to be at a 6:00 p.m. dinner engagement with family in a location one-half hour away. Let also assume that Hal has a list of errands and obligations that he would like to accomplish before his dinner engagement. Hal wants to purchase paint and supplies at a building supply store and bring the supplies home. He wants to work out at the fitness center for forty minutes, and he has six hours of work to do at his office.

Hal needs to work backwards from 6:00 p.m. First, since the dinner is one-half hour away and he wants to be sure to be on-time, he plans to leave his office for dinner at 5:15 p.m., leaving a fifteen-minute margin. Thus, he needs to start work at his office six hours earlier, or 11:15 a.m. His office is ten minutes from the fitness center, so he needs to leave the fitness center parking lot at 11:05. It takes him an hour and a quarter to get on the gym floor, work out, shower and dress. So he needs to arrive at the fitness center at 9:50. It takes him twenty minutes to drive from home to the fitness center, so he has to leave home at 9:30. He wants twenty minutes to unload his paint supplies and have a quick snack before departing for the fitness center, so he has to get home from the building supply store by 9:10. It is a fifteen-minute drive from the building supply store to home, so he must check out at the store by 8:55. He wants to leave thirty minutes to pick out his paint and supplies, so he must arrive at the building supply store by 8:25, and must leave home by 8:10. Hal likes to have an hour and a quarter to rise, stretch, dress and have a morning routine, so he must rise by 6:55 a.m. Thus, the night before, he resolves to get up by 6:55 a.m., and he assumes that if he does his errands in order, he will be fine.

Now, that is a lot of figuring. Moreover, unless you have practiced setting up an itinerary in this manner, you will probably get lost in the numbers several times before you get it sorted out. Try not to worry about that. With practice, you will improve. But, what about the problem with cognitive mapping? You will have to practice visualizing the various times in the itinerary. I have depicted one possibility on the next three pages.

Rise at 6:55

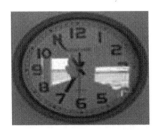

Leave for the building supply store at 8:10

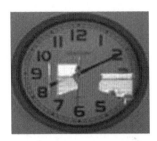

Arrive at the building supply store at 8:25

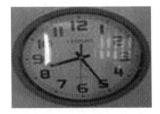

Check out at the building supply store at 8:55

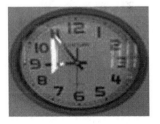

Arrive home to unload
supplies and get snack at 9:10

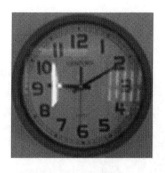

Leave home for the
fitness center at 9:30

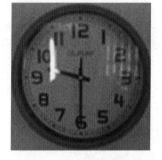

Arrive at fitness
Center at 9:50

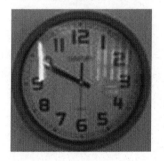

Leave fitness center for office at 11:05

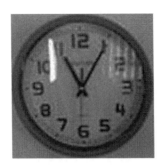

Arrive at office and start work at 11:15

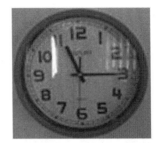

Leave office to go to family dinner at 5:15

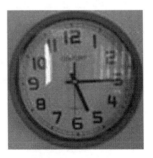

As previously stated, you will probably become lost with the times and numbers when you first attempt to set an itinerary by working backward from your end point. I have included the clocks in the previous illustration, as making a mental picture of a clock may assist you in keeping track of your obligations as you map them out in your mind. Nevertheless, this is a challenging task for persons with ADHD issues, so when you first experiment with itineraries, you will probably need to use pencil and paper.

It will take some practice for you to be able to make sufficiently accurate time predictions regarding travel times and times to accomplish errands. However, if you are able to practice the method and master it, it will be really worth it. You will not over schedule yourself. If you consider scheduling too many errands or activities, planning the itinerary will make it obvious to you that the itinerary will not work. You will make adjustments and will end up with a realistic itinerary. You will be much more relaxed and happy during your day, knowing that you will meet your obligations. And, of utmost importance, you will feel clever and masterful rather than disorganized and inept.

—■—

CHAPTER 28
Method Eighteen
Do a Trick With Arithmetic

———

You are going to encounter arithmetic problems
in your life, whether you want to or not.

THROUGHOUT THIS BOOK, I HAVE been emphasizing certain concepts. For one, I have emphasized the point that persons with ADHD or ADHD-like issues often see their worlds as an array of complicated situations and obligations. For another, I have asserted that organizing any one part of a person's life and experience can serve as a catalyst – as a rallying point around which other parts of life may also become organized. You may recall that I illustrated this point by describing the way in which, when ice freezes, a chaotic array of water molecules organizes itself around the first hexagonal ice crystal.

You are going to encounter arithmetic problems in your life, whether you want to or not. You may reach the checkout cashier at your favorite store, wondering whether you are being charged the correct price on an item that is on sale. You may dine in a restaurant and have difficulty computing a fifteen or twenty percent tip. You may be negotiating the purchase of a new car, and find yourself wondering whether the monthly payment being quoted makes sense in terms of the purchase price of the car. If you have difficulty making these arithmetic calculations, this will add to your sense that your world is full of impossible complications. If, on the other hand, you have learned some tricks to make these calculations, you will have a sense of mastery, with increased self-esteem, and your world will feel more manageable.

In addition, you may recall that in the section on cognitive mapping I made the point that persons with ADHD may have some problems with basic arithmetic. I believe that this problem has at its origins a difficulty visualizing numbers on a number line. I illustrated this point by describing the difficulty many individuals have when I ask them to subtract 68 from 73. These same persons have no difficulty telling me that three sheep on the right of a fence and two sheep on the left of the fence add up to five sheep.

Michael Von Aster and Ruth Shalev describe "number sense'" as "a term denoting the ability to represent and manipulate numerical magnitude nonverbally on an internal number line." If a child in the early school years cannot visualize numbers in various ways, including seeing them on a number line, that child will struggle to perform well in basic arithmetic. This will lead the child to feel anxiety when being taught arithmetic, and the anxiety will lead to more poor performance, and so forth. This is our "old friend" the positive feedback loop, or vicious cycle.

What can you do if your child is struggling in arithmetic? Here is a method you may want to consider. Acquire a big supply of chalk, and find a place where there is a large, flat area of asphalt. You may find such an area in a school playground, beside a supermarket or in the corner of a big mall parking lot. Using your chalk, draw a long line. Draw crosshatches on the line, approximately one-foot apart - one crosshatch for each number. Make the crosshatches bold for multiples of FIVE, and make them very bold for multiples of TEN. Thus, there will be ten feet between zero and ten, ten feet between ten and twenty, et cetera. A beanbag or two will be helpful.

Next, play a game with your child. Ask your child to stand on the number zero. Place a beanbag on ten and ask your child to walk from zero to ten, counting aloud as s/he goes. Do the same thing from ten to twenty. Try the same thing for five to fifteen and from fifteen to twenty-five. Your child will be getting the idea of the numerical distance between multiples of ten and five. Try little addition and subtraction problems, each time asking your child to move physically from place to place and to count aloud as s/he goes. Your child will be processing the information three ways: visually by seeing the number line, kinesthetically by moving from number to number, and through the language/auditory channel by counting aloud. There are those who believe that neurological development can be enhanced with appropriate training. Michael Von Aster and Ruth Shalev write, "a growing working memory enables neuroplastic development of an expanding mental number line during school years."

Ask your child to stand on the number twenty, and place beanbags on the numbers twenty-three and eighteen. Ask your child to subtract eighteen from twenty-three. Have him step from twenty-three to eighteen, one number at a time. Make sure s/he can see the numbers twenty-three and eighteen, and can see, feel and count the distance between them. A pad and pencil will help at this point. Write out the subtraction problem:

$$
\begin{array}{r}
23 \\
- \underline{18}
\end{array}
$$

If your child hesitates, go back to your chalk line and show him the numbers twenty-three and eighteen once again on the line. Then return to the pad and paper. Go back and forth between the physical number line and the pad and pencil until your child can see the written numerals and understand them in terms of the number line.

Next, work on numbers that are more than ten apart. That is, place bean bags on eighteen and thirty-three, and have your child step one number at a time from eighteen to thirty-three. Then, with pad and pencil, write out the subtraction problem:

$$\begin{array}{r} 33 \\ -\ \underline{18} \end{array}$$

You are trying at this point to de-mystify numbers that are farther apart, by using your child's newly enhanced understanding of tens. Thirty-three minus eighteen is not much more complicated than twenty-three minus eighteen when you understand tens.

Use your imagination and devise ways of using the number line to help your child gain familiarity with numbers, and confidence in his/her ability to handle them. Once your child gains some confidence in this area, s/he will experience less anxiety, and improved performance, in school when arithmetic skills are taught. In addition, perhaps improved performance in arithmetic, and the improved confidence and self-esteem that accompanies it, will lead to improvement in other areas as well.

—■—

CHAPTER 29
Method Nineteen
Don't Shade Your Eyes - Subitize

If you have learned anything from this book, you have learned that your author believes that improved skill, organization or efficiency in any one domain of functioning has the potential to enhance other related functional areas as well.

D r. David Mills writes

"Subitizing is the innate ability to know, from a brief glance, how many of a small number of objects there are. Human babies can do this from birth, and this ability is shared with all primates. Subitizing is the first math ability and forms the basis for much -- perhaps all -- math ability that follows it."

Most persons can ascertain the number of objects up to five with relative ease, and some persons can succeed with up to nine objects, albeit with some reduced accuracy.

The ability to subitize is instrumental in many other functions besides its utility for mathematics. Burkhart Fischer states, "The capacity for subitizing contributes to reading, because it allows us to know how many letters are in a word without having to count them."

If you have learned anything from this book, you have learned that your author believes that improved skill, organization or efficiency in any one domain of functioning has the potential to enhance other related functional areas as well. From a phenomenological point of view, persons with ADHD or ADHD-like issues often experience a lack of clarity, or even some confusion, when looking out at their phenomenological field. That field may be a field of physical objects; persons with various roles; tasks or obligations; or concepts. Regardless of the content of the phenomenological field, it can be more difficult to grasp for persons with ADHD.

If we improve our ability to ascertain the number of objects in a group, are we not, at a basic level, improving our ability to comprehend our phenomenological field? Recall the sense convergence method. In that technique we reduced all the stimulation of the world to the single sound of a thermos bottle filling, and simultaneously reduced our responses to the world to the single action of turning off a tap. When we attained a smooth enjoyable sense of the coordination between input and output, we were able to bring that coordination with us to more complicated situations. Perhaps improving our ability to subitize is one more skill that we can bring with us in our attempt to comprehend our complex world and to relate more effectively to it.

Complex computer programs have reportedly been developed to work on improving the ability to subitize. However, very simple methods may also be used. Play a little game with a bottle of vitamin pills. Hold the bottle of vitamin pills, with the cap off, in one hand. Shake a small number of pills into the palm of your other hand and make an immediate decision as to how many pills are there. Count them to check your accuracy. Perform this game a number of times, and see if your skill improves. Next, look for opportunities to practice this skill a few times per day in your day-to-day life. If you see a small group of children playing, make a quick calculation of the number of children, and then count to check your accuracy. There will be an endless supply of situations in which you may practice this skill. By practicing the skill of subitizing, you are exercising the capacity of your eyes and brain to apprehend a selection of objects in your world. You are learning to create a small amount of order from a small amount of chaos.

Eleanor Maguire and associates used structural MRI to study the brains of London Taxi drivers. London is a city laid out in a particularly complex way, and learning to navigate it successfully requires acquisition of large amounts of visual-spatial data. Maguire reported,

> Hippocampal volume correlated with the amount of time spent as a taxi driver (positively in the posterior and negatively in the anterior hippocampus). These data are in accordance with the idea that the posterior hippocampus stores a spatial representation of the environment and can expand regionally to accommodate elaboration of this representation in people with a high dependence on navigational skills. It seems that there is a capacity for local plastic change in the structure of the healthy adult human brain in response to environmental demands.

The human brain can change, adapt and grow in response to various demands. Learning to subitize may seem to be a trivial task in comparison to learning to navigate the streets of London. However, we know that our brains have the capacity to adapt to new demands. This should give us hope and confidence. Practicing new ways to organize our perceptions and our behavior does in fact have the potential to improve our skills in navigating our world in a more efficient, effective and successful manner.

—■—

CHAPTER 30
Method Twenty
The Good Conduct Self Award

———

We are not totally defined by our shortcomings.
Therefore, I am suggesting that you take some
time every day – at least three times per day – to
remind yourself of some of your good qualities.

WE ALL HAVE WEAKNESSES OR shortcomings. We have all been subjected to criticism by others, and at times we all subject ourselves to self-criticism. This method applies to many different situations. For instance, if you have ADHD or ADHD-like issues, you have probably heard people say things to you such as:

- You are such a space shot!
- Why can't you be on time?
- Finish what you are doing before jumping to something else!
- Will you please stay focused on what we are doing here!

And you probably subject yourself to similar criticism. The problem is that criticism – either by yourself or by others – will cause you to feel discouraged. Moreover, discouragement will reduce rather than strengthen your ability to improve.

If you value living as effectively, efficiently and successfully as you reasonably can, it is important that you address your shortcomings and strive to improve. Your ability to improve will be stronger if you maintain your self-esteem. We are not totally defined by our shortcomings. Therefore, I am suggesting that you take some time every day – at least three times per day – to remind yourself of some of your good qualities. I am suggesting that you give yourself a frequent "good conduct self-reward."

Please look at the following list of positive qualities. Then, make a selection of three-to-five of these qualities that meet the following criteria:

1. You believe this is one of your qualities.
2. You believe this is an important attribute.
3. You are proud of yourself for possessing this quality.

Active	artistic	bright	caring
cheerful	clever	considerate	courageous
courteous	creative	dutiful	employed
forgiving	friendly	funny	generous
gentle	helpful	honest	industrious
intelligent	kind	likeable	loving
loyal	open	patient	practical

reasonable	respectful	responsible	resourceful
sober	thrifty	thoughtful	trustworthy

Of course, you do not have to restrict yourself to the thirty-six qualities I have listed. Use any positive quality that you think is important, that you possess, and of which you are proud.

Next, I want you to make a memory device to help you remember the three to five positive qualities you have chosen. I have helped many patients devise such memory devices in session. If you can, create a word, or acronym, using the first letters of each of your chosen qualities. For example, if you have chosen artistic, dutiful and patient, you could use the acronym "PAD":

- P - patient
- A - artistic
- D - dutiful

If you have chosen courteous, intelligent, kind, respectful and thoughtful, you could create the acronym "TRICK":

- T - thoughtful
- R - respectful
- I - intelligent
- C - courteous
- K - kind

Train yourself to know your memory device as well as you know your date of birth. And, train yourself to remind yourself of your chosen three-to-five positive qualities frequently. Remember:

- Living effectively, efficiently and productively is a worthwhile goal.
- You may have to address your issues or shortcomings to improve.
- Maintaining your self-esteem will reduce discouragement and will increase your motivation to do well. Remember our discussion of negative feedback loops. If you have a period of reduced efficiency and reduced self-esteem, let it be a signal to strengthen your use of the methods you have learned here, including the good conduct self reward.

———

CHAPTER 31
A Day in the Life: Success Coping with ADHD

———

MEGAN IS A HYPOTHETICAL INDIVIDUAL who has recovered from ADHD by using the methods presented in this book. Let us follow her as she proceeds through a day in her life. Megan awakens and rises at 6:00 a.m. She is due at work at 9:00, and she hopes to get a few things done before then. She wants to work out at the gym, stop at the drugstore for a few items and go to the post office for stamps.

At first, Megan has no idea how much she can do and what her schedule will look like. She recalls the "planning effective itinerary" method and applies it. She needs to leave the drugstore by 8:45 to be at work before 9:00, and she needs ten minutes to shop. She therefore needs to arrive at the drugstore by 8:35. The drugstore is ten minutes from the fitness center, so she would need to leave the fitness center by 8:25. She needs twenty minutes to shower and dress, so she has to get off the exercise floor by 8:05, after a forty-minute workout that would start by 7:25. She needs to leave twenty-five minutes to drive to the fitness center, get into her gym outfit and get onto the exercise floor. Thus, she needs to leave the house at 7:00. She needs an hour for a comfortable morning routine between rising and leaving home. The post office errand is obviously out for this morning, but she now has an idea of her morning itinerary.

Megan starts her morning routine by making her bed and dressing. Then she briefly runs into a snag. She knows she has to pack her gym bag, have a quick breakfast, pack a lunch, and put a few files into the shoulder bag that she brings to work. She is suspended among these tasks, and is momentarily immobilized. She remembers the stop-scan-do method and immediately applies it. A quick scan of her tasks tells her that her breakfast should come first. Next, she stops, scans and decides to pack her lunch while she is still in the kitchen. Again, she stops and scans, and decides the gym bag can be packed while she is upstairs getting the files she needs. Putting the files in the shoulder bag is thus the last of the four tasks.

Megan notices it is 6:50, and she has ten minutes before she has to leave. As she looks around her home, she is uncomfortable with the clutter she sees. She has no time for thorough housekeeping, but remembers the "Do Ten Things" method, and decides to apply it. She sees yesterday's newspaper on the coffee table, puts it in the recycle bin and says "one." A throw pillow is on the floor, so she tosses it on the sofa and says "two." A jacket is draped over the arm of the sofa, and she hangs it in the closet and says "three." She proceeds in this manner until she has done ten quick tasks, sees that the house looks better, and she is ready to leave.

However, she has had episodes of leaving with the heat still running, forgetting her lunch, et cetera, so she utilizes the "acronym for remembering" method. Her acronym is "CLASP," which stands for comb, lunch, air conditioner (or heat), shoulder bag and purse. She checks these five items, turns down the heat, and is out the door at five minutes before eight.

A half-hour later Megan is striding along on a treadmill at the fitness center. She is feeling okay physically, but she has the nagging sensation that she is forgetting something. She cannot put her finger on it, so she employs the "Internal Monitoring Method" (Mr. Ship).

M   Material, financial
R   Recreational, physical
S   Social and family
H   Home, domestic
I   Intellectual, spiritual
P   Professional

When she gets to the "S" for social and family, she suddenly remembers her bother's birthday is coming soon, and she has not yet bought a card. She has been trying to strengthen her relationship with her brother and wants to be sure to get a card sent to him on time. That was what was nagging at her. Nonetheless she proceeds to the last three initials and, when she gets to professional, she recalls that she needs 3X5" cards and pens for the office. She had already planned to stop at the drugstore for paper towels and dish soap, but now she has five items to purchase.

Megan used to often leave stores without having remembered to buy something, and it made her feel disorganized. She decides to apply the "Method of Loci." She will use the first five places in the list of ten typical places that a high school student will visit on a school day. The first five places are: getting out of bed, the bathroom, the bedroom closet, the breakfast table, and the bus stop. She imagines waking up and seeing a giant birthday card at the foot of her bed. She imagines going to the bathroom and finding paper towel instead of bathroom tissue. She imagines going to the bedroom closet and slipping on some 3X5" cards on the floor. She imagines going to the breakfast table and finding a cereal bowl full of pens. Last, she imagines waiting for a school bus and seeing a giant bottle of dish soap in the bicycle rack on the front of the bus. She is now confident that these images will help her remember all of the five items.

When Megan is at the drugstore, she has found four items and is looking for her favorite style of pens. There is a vast sea of pens in front of her. Her eyes begin to dart about, making her start to feel tense and scattered. But, she recalls the "Gentle Eye Sweep Method." She starts at the top left and sweeps her eyes to the right along the top row of pens. Not finding hers, she drops her eyes to the next level and begins to sweep her eyes back to the left. Midway through that sweep, she finds her pens, with ease and in a relaxed manner.

Megan arrives at her parking space a few minutes before nine o'clock. She is eager to get into the office and is about to jump out of the car. Then she remembers "RCA-Victor" – relax, complete what you are doing, attend to what you need next, and velocity (go). She uses her brief relaxation method (she takes a slow, deep breath and thinks "calm" as she exhales, focusing on a sense of letting go, and on a sense of stillness, like a pond without a ripple). As she looks around to see that she has "completed" what she needs to do before getting out of the car, she sees her keys in the ignition. "That was a close call," she thinks, as she takes the keys. Locking her keys in her car would have been both inconvenient and embarrassing. She gathers her purse, puts the pens and 3X5" cards in to the shoulder bag, locks the car and heads for the office.

Megan arrives in her office, puts down her purse and shoulder bag, and finds herself feeling a sense of tension and impatience about starting her day. She pauses, does her Brief Relaxation Method, and begins her day in a more moderate state of arousal.

Eight hours later, Megan has completed a busy workday, and is eager to get back home. She looks around her office and sees that there are many file folders, papers and other paraphernalia lying about. She pauses and thinks. She does not want to take the time to put everything away, but if she leaves it the way it is, she may have a difficult time finding things tomorrow. Then she recalls the "60 / 40 Principle." She realizes that if she files sixty percent of the folders and papers that are lying about, the remaining forty percent will not be difficult to manage tomorrow. Therefore, she clears up a little more than half the mess and departs.

While driving home, Megan finds the cars in front of her have suddenly bunched up and slowed down, and she has to apply her brakes quickly and hard. She barely stops in time. Megan remembers the "Sense Convergence Method." While practicing with a thermos bottle, she has learned to coordinate her responses to the world with the stimulation coming in. She applies the method to her drive home. She watches the line of traffic up ahead. As soon as the space between cars narrows, or as soon as she sees a brake light going on, she lightens up on the gas pedal. The rest of the drive home is comfortable, safe and without incident.

Fifteen minutes later Megan pulls into her driveway. Before getting out of the car, she thinks about the day that has passed. She feels that she has been competent, clever, well organized and efficient. She has not always felt that way, and is much happier now. Before getting out of her car, she uses the method of giving herself a "Good Conduct Award." Her mnemonic device is "REACH":

R   reasonable
E   employed
A   active
C   clever
H   honest

She reviews the positive attributes that she feels are true of her. In particular, she thinks about how well she handled her day, compared to the way in which she would have handled it prior to learning the methods she employed today. Thus, she especially feels clever.

On the following page is a chart describing the twelve situations Megan encountered, the methods she employed, and the nature of the difficulties she managed to avoid.

Situation Encountered	Method Employed	Difficulties and Inconveniences Avoided
Rising in a.m.	Itinerary	Overscheduling, with resulting anxiety and lateness
Getting ready in a.m.	Stop-scan-do	Feeling disorganized, scattered and inefficient.
5-minutes before leaving home	Do 10 Things	Return to a cluttered house, with feelings of inefficiency and failure
Departure	Acronym for Remembering	Major inconvenience of arriving at work without needed belongings.
Treadmill	Internal Monitoring	Forgetting brother's birthday, with loss of opportunity to rebuild that relationship. Lack of needed supplies at work.
Challenge of remembering items needed for purchase	Method of Loci	Forgotten items, with resulting negative self-statements about inefficiency.

Shopping at Drug-store	Gentle Eye Scan	Feelings of tension and of being scattered while searching tor item on shelf.
Arrival at work	RCA-V	Major inconvenience of locking self out of vehicle.
Office	Brief Relaxation	Beginning day with tension, which could have led to errors, impatience or irritability with others.
End of day	The 60 / 40 Principle	Next day could have begun with disarray, inconvenience and self-recrimination
Driving on highway	Sense Convergence	Injury or death
Arriving home	Good Conduct Reward	Missed opportunity to feel good about self

In one day, Megan has utilized twelve of the twenty methods described in this book. Moreover, not one of the methods required her to consult a calendar, write a list, enlist the help of another person, or use an electronic reminder. She has managed to avoid difficulties and to enjoy an organized, efficient day strictly with internal skills. She has built habits that sustain her effectiveness. Perhaps her use of these methods has resulted in structural changes in the brain, as suggested in research by Bogdan Draganski and many others. Alternatively, perhaps her use of the methods has resulted in functional changes in the brain (effective synapses, myelination, or neurotransmitter activity) as suggested by Dietsje Jolles. Regardless of the exact explanation, by mastering the methods described, Megan has essentially trained her brain to be more efficient, and her life is improved. I encourage you to learn to use the methods that have been provided. Your life can improve as well.

—◼—

References

Faraone Biederman, "Current concepts on the neurology of ADHD," *Journal of Attention Disorders*, 2002, 6 (1), pp. 7-16.

Kumar Budur et al, "Non-stimulant treatment for ADHD," *Psychiatry*, July 2005, 2 (7), pp. 44-58.

Diagnostic and Statistical Manual of Mental Disorders, Fourth Edition, Washington, DC: American Psychiatric Association, 2007.

Diagnostic and Statistical Manual of Mental Disorders, Fifth Edition, Arlington, VA: American Psychiatric Association, 2013.

Bogdan Draganski et al,"Temporal and spatial dynamics of brain structure changes during extensive learning," *Journal of Neuroscience*, 2006:26 (23) pp. 6314-6317.

Fisher, Burkhart, "Subitizing dymanic vision, saccade and fixation control in dyslexia," in John Stein, editor, *Visual Aspects of Dyslexia*, Oxford University Press, 2012.

Gillberg, Christopher, ADHD and its Many Associated Problems, New York: Oxford University Press, 2014.

Groffman, Sidney, "Subitizing: Vision therapy for math deficits," Journal of Optimal Visual Development, 2009: 40 (4), pp. 229-238.

Britta Holzel et al, "Mindfulness practice leads to increases in regional brain gray matter density, *Psychiatry Research: Neuro Imaging,* 2011:191(1).

James Hudziak and Stephen Faraone, "Meta-analysis of genome-wide association studies of ADHD," *Journal of the American Academy of Child and Adolescent Psychiatry,* 2010: 49 (9), pp. 884-897.

Jensen, Peter S., "Current Concepts and Controversies in the Diagnosis and Treatment of ADHD," *Current Psychiatry Reports,* 2000, 2: 102-109.

Dietsje Jolles and Eveline Crone, "Training the developing brain: a neuro-cognitive perspective," in *Frontiers in Neuroscience,* Karbach and Schubert, editors

Kerstin Konrad and Simon Eckoff, "Is the ADHD brain wired differently? A review of structural and functional connectivity on attention deficit hyperactivity disorder." *Human Brain Mapping,* June 2010, Volume 31, Issue 6, pp. 904-916.

Dawei Li et al, "Meta-analysis shows significant association between dopamine system genes and ADHD," Human Molecular Genetics, Vol. 15 (14), pp. 2276-2284.

Durston, Sarah, "A review of the biological bases of ADHD: What have we learned from imaging studies?" *Mental Retardation and Developmental Disabilities Research Review,* 2003, Volume 9 (3), pp. 184-195.

Eleanor Maguire et al, "Navigation-related structural change in the hippocampi of London taxi drivers." *Proceedings of the National Academy of Sciences of the United Sates of America,* Volume 97, No. 8, pp. 4398-4403.

Jonathan Mill & Arturas Petronis, "Pre and peri-natal environmental risks for ADHD: the potential role of epigenetic processes in mediating susceptibility," *Child Psychology and Psychiatry,* 2008: 49 (10), pp. 1020-1030.

Moalem, Sharon, *Survival of the Sickest,* 2007: Harper Collins.

Sandeep Ravindram, "Barbara McClintock and the discovery of jumping genes," *Proceedings of the National Academy of Sciences of the United States,* Vol. 109 (50), pp. 2198-20199.

Rubia, Katya et al, "Abnormal brain activation during inhibition and error detection in medication-naïve adolescents with ADHD," *American Journal of Psychiatry,* 2005, Volume 166: pp. 1067-1075.

Safren, Steven A. et al, "Cognitive-behavioral therapy for ADHD in medication-treated adults with continued symptoms," in *Behaviour Research and Therapy,* 2005, 43: 7 pp. 831-842.

Saul, Richard, MD, *ADHD Does Not Exist,* New York: Harper Collins, 2014.

Mark Sciutto and Miriam Eisenberg, "Evaluating the evidence for and against the over diagnosis of ADHD," *Journal of Attention Deficit,* 11 (2), pp. 106-113.

P. Shaw, K. Eckstrand et al, "Attention deficit hyperactivity disorder is characterized by a delay in cortical maturation," in *Proceedings of the*

National Academy of Sciences of the USA, Volume 104, Number 49, pp. 19649-19654.

Shue, Karen and Douglas, Virginia, "Attention deficit hyperactivity disorder and the frontal lobe syndrome," in *Brain and Cognition*, Volume 20, Issue 1, pp. 104-124.

Gail Tripp and Jeff Wickens, "Dopamine transfer deficit: a neurological theory of altered reinforcement mechanisms in ADHD," *Journal of Child Psychology and Psychiatry*, 2008, Volume 49, pp. 691-704.

U.S. Department of Health and Human Services, National Institutes of Health, NIH Publication No. 12-3572, Revised 2012.

Michael Von Aster and Ruth Shalev, "Number development and developmental dyscalculia," *Developmental Medicine and Child Neurology*, 2007: 49 (11), pp. 868-873.

Yale University School of Medicine, "Fundamentals of ADHD: circuits and pathways," *The Journal of Clinical Psychiatry* [2006, 67 Suppl 8:7-12].

—■—

About the Author

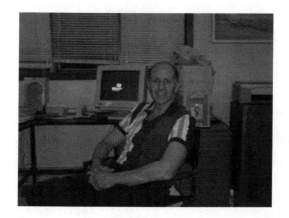

D R. MICHAEL SLAVIT IS A psychologist in private practice. Dr. Slavit received his Bachelor's degree from Brown University, his Master's from the University of Rhode Island and his Ph.D. from the University of Texas at Austin. He is board certified in Cognitive and Behavioral Psychology, but he believes his most important credential is the confidence his patients have in him.

Dr. Slavit is the author of *Cure Your Money Ills: Improve Your Self-esteem through Personal Budgeting, Your Life: An Owner's Guide* and *Lessons from Desiderata.* He has also written numerous handouts, brochures and "Ask the Psychologist" columns. You may visit Dr. Slavit's website: *MikeSlavit.com.*

89490026R00092

Made in the USA
Lexington, KY
29 May 2018